BODY LOVE

BODY LOVE

LIVE IN BALANCE, WEIGH WHAT
YOU WANT, AND FREE YOURSELF
FROM FOOD DRAMA FOREVER

KELLY LeVEQUE

wm

WILLIAM MORROW

An Imprint of HarperCollins*Publishers*

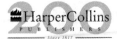

This book contains advice and information relating to health care. It should be used to supplement rather than replace the advice of your doctor or another trained health professional. If you know or suspect you have a health problem, it is recommended that you seek your physician's advice before embarking on any medical program or treatment. All efforts have been made to assure the accuracy of the information contained in this book as of the date of publication. This publisher and the author disclaim liability for any medical outcomes that may occur as a result of applying the methods suggested in this book.

HarperCollins books may be purchased for educational, business, or sales promotional use. For information, please e-mail the Special Markets Department at SPsales@harpercollins.com.

FIRST EDITION

Photos by Vanessa Tierney

Graphics by Amber Moon

Designed by Bonni Leon-Berman

Library of Congress Cataloging-in-Publication Data has been applied for.

ISBN 978-0-06-256914-1

19 20 21   SCP   20 19 18

I dedicate this book to my husband, Chris—my soul mate,

the yin to my yang, my best friend, and my perfect partner in life.

CONTENTS

Contents

FOREWORD

THE DESIRE TO LIVE the healthiest, most sustainable life that I could is what led me to challenge the status quo and start The Honest Company. And when I met Kelly, I knew I had found a kindred spirit. We connected in 2015, at a time when I was struggling with a few health issues (inflammation being one of them) and just not feeling my best. And, like most women, I wanted to drop a few pounds. Los Angeles has no shortage of nutritionists, health gurus, and wellness experts, but Kelly had worked wonders for one of my best friends, so instinct told me that she was special.

During our first meeting, I peppered Kelly with all sorts of questions (it's who I am, I want to know *why*) and quickly realized we were operating on the same wavelength. She's a geek for the science behind what we eat and the products we use, just like me. And as we dug through my pantry, dissected my typical grocery list and went through a "day-in-the-life" of what I was eating, she explained things in clear, simple terms, armed me with practical advice, and infused me with a renewed sense of confidence. It's one of the best things about Kelly: she sets you up for self-sustaining success.

Naturally, when I heard she was putting her knowledge and her approach into a book, I was thrilled. Not only because I've had such incredible results working with her, but because I believe in who she is, what she does, and how she does it. She's passionate about her work, dedicated to helping others, conscientious of different lifestyles and always, always, always a spark of positive energy in my life.

And *Body Love* as a title? Killer. How many of us fall out of love with our bodies, our curves, and even ourselves? Believe me, as an actress, I've felt the pressure we all feel (times a thousand) to be *this* weight or *that* jean size or have *those* legs. Sorry, but I don't like trying to fit some idealized notion of "perfection." I like me. My husband, Cash, likes me. And the funny thing is, once Kelly helped me let go of some of that pressure, the results I wanted—for me—came quickly and naturally (eleven inches in about six weeks!). It's amazing what a little knowledge, confidence, and body love can do.

At the heart of it, Kelly's approach aligns perfectly with my personal philosophy on food and nutrition. I call it honest eating, but really, it's just about eating clean, organic, and nutrient-dense food. What really clicked for me: Her simple explanation of the science behind it all—how the right amount of macronutrients (her "Fab Four") on my plate or in my smoothie will balance my blood sugar and hunger hormones. I also love what her approach *isn't*—it's not about rules, calorie counting, or bland, boring food.

Case in point: I like eating whatever I want (literally, whatever) one day a week. When I mentioned this to Kelly, she didn't judge or lecture me. There wasn't even the slightest bit of guilt. She just smiled and said, "I got you, girl, this isn't all or nothing." It was so refreshing and empowering to hear. Kelly gets it. She's a woman, she's been there, and she's got you, too.

XO Jessica Alba

INTRODUCTION

HELLO! I'M THRILLED YOU'VE picked up *Body Love* and want to *be well!* My name is Kelly LeVeque, and I can't wait to share with you my approach to clean eating, wellness, and weight loss—which was originally called Be Well By Kelly (or BWBK).

At its core, *Body Love* is about feeling *empowered,* not overwhelmed, by food and nutrition. It's about using **light, science-driven structure** to stay on course (and autocorrect, if necessary), not being chained to an unsustainable or overly restrictive diet. It's about learning simple tips and tricks to **eat to satiety** and **naturally** balance your hunger hormones, not fighting not to eat. It's about ditching the food drama. No more aggressive cleanses; no more frustrating do-not-eat lists; no more yo-yo-inducing fad diets.

Why is my approach so different from other diets out there? Because (a) it's not a diet, and (b) **it's not a diet.** It's a realistic, sustainable, twenty-first-century approach that is rooted in the science of human nutrition, and it achieves real results. Best of all, my approach puts the power in your hands, so you can eat the foods you love and build your own healthy lifestyle. So if you're here to feel empowered and liberated, you're in the right place. My approach is for you.

Cultural attitudes toward food, nutrition, and wellness are shifting. It's not just the focus of people who shop at Whole Foods and wear lululemon; whether they know it or not, most of the wider population is gravitating toward a more personalized, holistic approach. People care more than ever about what they eat, are more educated than ever about where it comes from and how it's made, and are more attuned than ever to how it affects them *personally*. Thankfully, most people are open-minded and willing to accept an important, nonnegotiable truth: that food has the power to shape not only our bodies and brains but also our lives and futures.

I wrote this book to help you understand how the foods you're eating are affecting you and why. I want you to look and feel great, whatever that means to you. I want you to set yourself up for personal food freedom, not just for the next trip where a bikini or bathing suit is required, but for the rest of your life.

In *Body Love*, you'll learn how to nourish your body with clean, whole foods that prevent elevated blood sugar, inflammation, and gut issues. You'll learn why certain foods make us gain weight and get sick and have the potential to create serious health problems. And I'll show you how certain foods can actually help you *lose* pounds and rediscover your optimal weight. One of the most powerful discoveries you'll make is that our bodies are not biologically designed to "diet." They're designed to be fed, to respond to real hunger signals, and to feel satisfied and energized by the foods we eat. No one is born to be sick, fat, or unhealthy. In fact, our bodies are designed and wired to **be well.**

My program will help you build light and sustainable structure from this biological blueprint. I'll also equip you with simple strategies and tools, such as the **Fab Four** (what I like to call protein, fat, fiber, and greens) and the **Fab Four Smoothie** (a go-to solution to get the Fab Four in one meal), to seamlessly apply this knowledge to your everyday life. You'll see and feel results because you'll be giving your body the food it wants, when it wants it. (It's smarter than you. It knows!)

My approach isn't simply about losing weight so you feel vibrant and sexy. It's a powerful state of mind that emerges when you give your body the nourishment it needs. It's confidence, peace of mind, and a way to let go of all that mental baggage. The right foods will invigorate you mentally and liberate you psychologically. When you eat this way, you'll feel full of energy and your brain will feel whip-smart. You'll stop worrying about food all the time and let go of food guilt, anxiety, and self-shame. You'll have the confidence to conquer any menu and trust yourself to make healthy choices because your body isn't craving sugar-laden junk.

The title of this book is *Body Love* for a reason. Loving your body means respecting it, understanding it, and listening to it. Yes—I'm absolutely devoted to clean eating, optimizing my health, and living a conscious life of wellness. But I also want a glass of rosé on a Friday, brunch with my girlfriends on a Sunday, and a summer vacation to decompress and recharge my batteries—all without worrying about "ruining a diet." I want to have my gluten-free cake and eat it too, without weight gain, inflammation, food guilt, and aging. I created my practice so I could ditch food drama and simply enjoy eating in a way that preserves good health and overall wellness, and that makes weight loss easy. Treating my body with this kind of flexibility with an eye on balance is the way I learned to truly love my body.

The genesis of my practice goes back to my time in high school. While the world was fretting about the sure-to-be-coming Y2K computer crash, I was trying to convince my girlfriends not to do the latest, sure-*not*-to-work crash diet. I was naturally drawn to the science of food and nutrition, and continued to pursue that knowledge passionately during my college years. My dad always encouraged me to go into business, so after graduation I paired business with my love of science and began an eight-year career in the medical field. I worked for Fortune 500 companies such as Johnson & Johnson, Stryker, and Hologic, and ended at Agendia in personalized medicine, offering tumor gene mapping and molecular subtyping to oncologists. Meanwhile, on the side, I gave a lot of free advice about food and nutrition to friends and family—how to stop the sugar-craving cycle that triggers binge eating, how to reduce bloating, how to lose five to fifteen pounds before a wedding, how to clear hormonal acne, how different foods affect pregnancy, and so on.

My career in medical science meant that I had to keep up with cutting-edge research on how diseases develop and how they can be treated. I loved the deep thinking required, especially the statistical analysis—deciphering data for statistical significance, distinguishing causation from correlation, and understanding why study design mattered so much. It was my job to then educate my clients (most of whom were MDs!) about how to integrate this latest research into their clinical practices so they could save lives. (In other words, I did what I do now! I read the research, deciphered its statistical significance, and educated my clients on research in a digestible way.) This skill helped me dig deeper into nutritional science, and the more I read, the more advice I gave to an ever-expanding group of people.

My interest in and passion for nutritional science grew naturally from this early immersion in medical science. I was fascinated by the line between wellness and disease, and was becoming especially drawn to the growing field of holistic nutrition. I finally decided to formalize my interest through training in integrative and clinical nutrition. After several years of eighteen-hour days (#hustle), working weekends (what's a weekend?), and balancing the demands of two jobs, I decided to strike out on my own and form a business that could help people stay healthy from the beginning. And so my business was born!

My work as a holistic nutritionist, health coach, and wellness expert has been the most gratifying, rewarding work of my life. Over the past four years, my client base has grown from a small, devoted group in Los Angeles to a global network of men and women who live to **be well**. My clientele runs the gamut. I work with men and women of all ages, from all sorts of backgrounds, who have a wide array of different health issues, goals, and lifestyle preferences. I've received a lot of positive attention because a good number of my clients are celebrities (actors, actresses, television personalities, and professional athletes), but I work with everyone: moms, dads, brides, grooms, vegans, vegetarians, lawyers and other professionals, executives, entrepreneurs, and so on. I also write articles and contribute to many well-known publications and blogs. All this has helped build a groundswell of support and interest in my approach.

But there are two even more powerful reasons that word has spread: my approach delivers **results,** and it's **realistic**.

What do I mean by results? For starters, anyone can lose four easy pounds in a week just by starting their day with one of the Fab Four Smoothies in this book (they start on page 140, if you want to take a peek). If you stick to this alone, you'll more than likely lose up to ten pounds in two and half weeks. You can also clear acne, manage polycystic ovarian syndrome (PCOS), and reverse diabetes and heart disease markers while you're at it. (You don't have to be overweight to be prediabetic, with elevated blood sugar and inflammation silently laying down the foundation for heart disease.)

And I love to hear from my clients that my approach is realistic. Why? Because it's a totally sustainable lifestyle that doesn't require overthinking, chaining yourself to eat-this-not-that lists, or a mandatory commitment to grueling workouts. You're not going to be made to carry around a list of foods you can or can't eat. You won't be told to eat every three to four hours. You're never going to think about dieting again!

Essentially, *Body Love* offers an approach to eating and being well that's all about simplifying decisions so you don't have to overthink your food choices. I'll show you how to spend just fifteen minutes shopping early in the week so you're set up to open your fridge, pick from a few basic but nutritious ingredients, and go for it—instant, satisfying, delicious meals! I'll also show you how to easily prepare for dinners out, weekends away, and a host of other real-life "what should I eat?" moments. If you have intolerances or allergies, I'll help you feel empowered, not inhibited, in spite of your body's reactions. And if you find yourself feeling out of balance or off course, I'll show you how to quickly and easily autocorrect, sans guilt. My approach is a drama- and anxiety-free lifestyle that works at home and on the go, to fit the way you live.

THE HEART OF THE FAB FOUR LIFESTYLE

At its heart, my approach is rooted in my love of and trust in science, as well as my desire to simplify complicated information for everyone, so that it is easily accessible and makes sense. **Specifically, my approach is based on the chemistry of controlling and maintaining optimal blood sugar balance, so that your body uses (1) proteins, fats, and carbohydrates (macronutrients), (2) vitamins and minerals (micronutrients), and (3) antioxidants (phytonutrients) in ways that allow you to eat to satisfaction, naturally turn off your "hunger" hormones, and still lose (or maintain) weight.** The science of how our blood sugar works, coupled with an emphasis on eating real, anti-inflammatory whole foods, is what separates my program from the quick-fix fads, diets, and other trendy low-carb plans.

Through blood sugar balance, you'll get all you need to be vibrant and arrive at your own ideal weight. You'll rediscover that food should be enjoyed, not stressed over, especially as we return to basic, clean foods in their natural form. When we take away processed ingredients, packaged meals, and snacks (if you're reading this, you aren't a toddler and you don't need snacks!) and once again let our taste buds and stomachs enjoy delicious protein, fat, fiber, and greens (the Fab Four) unsullied by harmful chemicals, we relearn how to eat the way we were meant to eat—to satiety.

Have you ever counted calories? It's awful. We won't be doing it. The vast majority of diets out there have relied upon the misleading notion that any kind of weight loss must be about limiting—calories, portions, or food groups. But that's just not the case. My approach is all about balance.

Here's some of what you can expect:

- Actress and CEO Jessica Alba, 35, lost 11 inches in 6 weeks.
- Actress Kate Walsh, 49, drinks Fab Four Smoothies for health and longevity.
- Model and actress Molly Sims, 43, got back to her pre-baby weight within 12 weeks.
- Actress and director Emmy Rossum, 30, lost pounds before her wedding.
- Bethany, 45, lost 10 pounds in 4 weeks, 3 inches around her waist and hips, and even 1 inch around each arm.
- Mariah, 36, cured her sugar cravings; toned her abs, legs, and arms; and cleared her acne.
- Abby, 27, lost 8 pounds in 2 weeks and went down 2 jean sizes.
- Emily, 31, lost 30 pounds in 3 months by simply having breakfast! She enjoyed a Fab Four Smoothie daily.

And the men?

- Connor Cook, 23, a quarterback for the Oakland Raiders, lost 6 percent body fat and gained 9 pounds of muscle to prepare for the NFL draft.
- Evan Peters, 29, and Ben Hardy, 25, clocked in at less than 10 percent body fat before filming *X-Men: Apocalypse*.

Introduction

- Chris, 52, lost 15 pounds in 6 weeks while still eating out with clients.
- John, 42, not only lowered his cholesterol but lost 8 pounds in a month.
- Scott, 35, an actor, didn't need to lose weight, but his soft belly was transformed when he tried and stuck to my plan.

On my program, you'll absolutely lose weight (if that's your desire), lose fat, increase lean muscle mass, and go down at least one size in jeans. Your hair will become thicker and shinier, your skin will clear up and take on a fresh glow, and your overall appearance will remarkably improve. On the inside, your body will adapt to this new inner balance by no longer swelling, gaining weight, or breaking out as easily as before. You will feel more energetic and sleep better, too.

Clients come to me because they're frustrated and tired of feeling so out of control with their health. They sense that there is a simpler way, and they're right. I offer them commonsense techniques to get rid of their self-doubt and anxiety about food, and connect them to their *why*—why they want to lose weight, get in shape, find balance, change their lifestyle, and feel healthier. I want to share all their successes with you!

I want to show you how to read your body's signals and reset your blood sugar so you can enjoy true inner balance, rather than just jump onto the next best thing or the latest fad diet. I want you to feel empowered without being overwhelmed. And I want you to build a sustainable plan that works for you in the long term. The Fab Four is the simplest structure to balance blood sugar, avoid inflammation, and nourish your body daily. It's an approach to eating that sets you free, so you can just live and **be well**.

Finally, *Body Love* will come with a healthy dose of me! I fully invest myself in every single client I have. I live to inspire and love helping clients tackle whatever health issue, goal, or lifestyle desire they may have. Through the plan in this book, I want to invest in you. I want you to thrive and **be well!**

IT'S UP TO YOU: HOW THIS BOOK WORKS

Okay, not to get all Tony Robbins on you, but there's a process here, and it involves both of us. First me, then you. So listen up!

I'll give you all the information—the science, the light structure, the tips, tricks, strategies, and tools—in a clear, simple, digestible way, so that it makes sense. You'll immediately see why my approach achieves results—because it creates a realistic, sustainable plan based on how your body actually works.

Then it's your turn. My approach is useful only if you put it to use! You have to want this empowering change for yourself. That's your starting point. From there, I'll show you the path to food freedom. I said it'd be seamless to apply my approach to your life, and I meant it. I'm not one to overthink or overcomplicate things. My approach is the exact same—less thinking, less obsessing, and more living!

Case in point: To start, all you need to do is have a Fab Four Smoothie or put together a quick #Fab4 meal. Both will balance your blood sugar and **keep you in balance** throughout the day. You'll have a lot of choices, a lot of different flavors. You won't have to do any calorie counting or portion sizing. You won't make long lists to take to the grocery store. You won't have to check a do-not-eat list under the restaurant table. And you won't be drinking only juice for three, five, or seven days straight.

In fact, when new clients arrive, I often pause on giving them a full download on the food science and take a bit of a shortcut. I welcome them, give them a sense of where they're heading (to the Land of Be Well and Be Plenty!), and simply suggest that for one week they start their day with a Fab Four Smoothie (the recipes start on page 140). Then I send them on their way. After just one week, I start getting texts such as these:

Introduction

"OMG, down 4 lbs and feeling good! I heart you so hard."

"Kel, why am I not hungry it's 1:30pm? I don't get it. LOL"

"I get it! What's next? How can I lose even more weight?"

These are real texts, and I have hundreds more. Throughout the book, you'll read lots of success stories (and a few more texts) that will inspire and motivate you. These stories will illustrate the science at work and the quick ways my clients lost weight, lowered cholesterol, cleared their skin, and addressed a number of other health, food, and nutrition issues. The key takeaway is that eating the right anti-inflammatory foods and balancing our blood sugar are highly effective ways to tackle our unique challenges. Of course, each of us is very different. The concept of "bio-individuality" is an important thread throughout the book, and you'll be asked to do numerous self-checks so you stay attuned to your body's specific responses, reactions, and needs.

Let's take a closer look at how the book is organized to set you up for success!

In **Part One: The Science Behind the Fab Four Formula**, you'll learn what foods our bodies need, what blood sugar is, and why balancing blood sugar is so important. I'll introduce you to the basics of the #Fab4 formula, which will balance your blood sugar and help you find your sweet spot of satiety, so that you not only feel fed throughout the day (no hangry cravings!) but also exist in a body-state that burns fat and gobbles up excess pounds. In addition, you'll learn why the diets you've tried have failed, and about the food sources that trigger fat storage, bloating, sugar cravings, and precursors to disease. I'll also debunk some myths about fruit (too much sugar, even if they have fiber!), juicing (insulin resistance waiting to happen!), and gluten (going gluten-free isn't a fad!). You'll then respond to several questionnaires so that you become more aware of your body, its habits and reactions, and your tendencies and patterns.

In **Part Two: The Fab Four Solution**, I'll share an approach to eating that will free you from ever having to diet again. You'll learn exactly how eating meals based on the Fab Four set you up to lose weight and maintain that weight loss. You'll learn how to make the mental shift so you stop counting calories, let go of the restrictive deprivation mind-set that you associate with diets and weight loss, and replace it with a strong, confident, and very chill state of mind. You'll also respond to a few more questions and do a couple of exercises that will help you build your own lifestyle and make this shift real and life-lasting.

You'll also put pen to paper and clarify your goals—for the next week, month, and hopefully beyond—and start a Fab Four Notebook. Your notebook will also be a place where you can track your emotions related to food. It's not exactly a food diary, but an exercise that will be a huge help on your journey to food freedom. I am a big believer in the power of being conscious and honest with ourselves. It's not about perfection. It's about becoming aware of and truly connected to *you*—with all your questions, victories, mistakes, and corrections. My approach is designed to help you understand what works best for *you*, so you learn to be with yourself and trust yourself. I want you to own your process each and every day. Don't judge it, just be aware of it. The benefits, the bumps, the beauty, and the bliss—they're all part of **being well.**

In **Part Three: Your Fab Four Life**, I'll pull together the troubleshooting and other lifestyle advice that will ensure your success. You'll learn how to remove the drama from lunch and dinner and how to "autocorrect" after a weekend of fun, and if you have specific health conditions such as prediabetes or celiac disease, you can also learn how to use a glucometer (blood sugar monitor) to keep even more careful track of your blood sugar. By understanding how to adjust your eating when traveling, during the workday, and on vacation, you'll discover flexible solutions on the go.

You'll also discover how to maximize the effects of a minimal workout. Say good-bye to a mandatory seven-day-a-week workout regime! (Unless of course you love to move—in that case, more power to you. Just remember to rest!) I'll share a collection of cardio and strengthening exercises that will increase your insulin sensitivity, tone your body, and calm your mind. Chapters on all-over body vibrancy, managing stress, and beauty will help you create tools to support your new lifestyle. You'll find some fun tips for integrating meditation into your day and how to detox and use supplements to boost weight loss or keep you right where you want to be.

My approach is about discovering a livable, sustainable way of eating that makes you feel good and look great, whatever that means to you. Together, these simple steps will reset the biochemistry behind your metabolism and enable you to lose weight (if you want to), and feel and be healthier. I can't emphasize enough how good you will feel when you simply learn how to balance your blood sugar! From this place of calm and clarity, you'll learn to trust yourself. You'll learn how to stop doubting and overthinking your food choices. You won't worry about the number on the scale. You will simply be.

Remember: (a) This isn't a diet, and (b) **this isn't a diet!**

So let's get started!

PART ONE

THE SCIENCE BEHIND THE FAB FOUR FORMULA

1

ALL DIETS WORK . . . UNTIL THEY DON'T

AT THE OUTSET, LET'S get one thing straight: I've been there.

I've cried with my clothes piled around me because "nothing fits." I've tried to ditch ten pounds post-breakup and pre-vacation. I've had one too many glasses of wine and rebounded into a juice cleanse to compensate. At times I've felt helpless, unhappy with my body, and totally confused about what to do. I'm not the doctor giving you the miracle diet that fixes everyone. Nor am I the rigid eater who can easily say no to food. I'm an emotional human being and I've been on the roller coaster. I've been there—*everywhere*—with food, diets, and trying to be healthy.

As a young woman growing up in the 1990s and 2000s, when fad diets and health trends really burst into popular culture, I found myself devouring every health, diet, and lifestyle book I could find. I have always been active and healthy, with no serious medical conditions, but as many of you can probably relate, I was constantly striving for "perfection." Why is it that we're never satisfied? Like so many young women, I seemed to never stop wanting to be physically "better" somehow—a size smaller, with six-pack abs and a thigh gap, and always five pounds lighter (no matter my weight at the time). By high school, a third of my meals were salads. Sound familiar? I know I'm not alone in that kind of fixation on food, and it wasn't because of how I was raised.

I grew up in a stable, loving household. My parents were affectionate and supportive. I am the eldest of three girls, and my dad always told us that we were beautiful no matter what. My parents didn't obsess about food. Neither of them was a "food cop." In fact, the opposite was true. Our cabinets contained every packaged snack Costco sold—Wheat Thins, Goldfish, frosted animal crackers, and powdered doughnuts, to name a few. My mom made all our lunches, and we rarely went out for dinner. We had regular taco nights, pasta with meat sauce, pork chops with applesauce, and casseroles (my dad loves casseroles!). For lunch, I ate tuna salad, turkey sandwiches, cut-up cheese and apples, and chicken noodle soup. My food upbringing was a little slice of Americana, plain and simple.

But I had absorbed our culture's obsession with weight and perfection. So when I saw my weight fluctuate (which drove me crazy), I did what any thirteen-year-old going on thirty would do—I voraciously read diet books. My mom would say, "It's okay, honey. We grow out before we grow up." But I wanted to know more and find a solution. Some of the diets described in these books are ones you've probably heard of: Atkins, the Zone, South Beach, Mediterranean, blood type, alkaline, vegan. (Why I was allowed to fixate over diet books but not allowed to watch *The Simpsons* still baffles me.)

With every book and every year that passed, my insatiable desire and curiosity for the science of human nutrition and the body grew. And a funny thing also started to happen—the more I learned, the less I cared about the scale or being perfect, whatever "perfect" was. Why? Because I was beginning to understand *my* body, not some idealized version I saw on TV or in magazines. I also began to understand exactly what to do to feel in balance, get back on track if I didn't (or if I went to a party), and leave my meltdowns in the rearview mirror.

During my first few jobs out of college working for medical companies, I sought out research articles, combed through the primary sources on nutrition, and read specialty books like *Gut and Psychology Syndrome, Gluten Freedom,* and *Lights Out: Sleep, Sugar, and Survival.* Eventually my knowledge bucket spilled over and I found myself at parties talking to friends about what I was reading, what I was learning, and the benefits I was seeing. (Nerd alert!)

One of my first insights was this: When you look at a diet book, strip the title, and review the plan and approved foods, you'll see a lot of the same stuff repackaged with minor tweaks. Did you know that even the new Weight Watchers SmartPoints increase points for sugar and decrease points for protein? It's very similar to the Atkins, Mediterranean, and South Beach diets, with more counting and a bonus support group. Then came the gluten-free, high-fat, gut health, and lifestyle diets (such as Paleo and Whole30), and the same was true.

So what are they all really saying? Eat vegetables, healthy fats, and wild proteins. And how are people losing weight, calming inflammation, and feeling great? The exact same way! The best diet books work because they're based on how our bodies metabolize food, which I'm all for. But at the same time, many of them cause food anxiety, diet addiction, and low self-esteem. Because they're diets!

Over time, I became more and more confident that I knew how to eat in a way that would make me feel good. I committed to living a clean lifestyle and eating in a healthy way, without obsessing about food. And eventually, the desire to "eat healthy" converged with my intellectual curiosity to know more about how the things we eat affect our health, wellness, and emotional well-being. In forming my company, I'd finally caught up to what I was always meant to be doing. (My college transcript will show that the best grade I received at USC was in my Nature of Human Health and Disease class.) Like no other subject, the science of nutrition and biology is catalogued in my brain. My inner librarian is on point—I can still easily reference and compare new studies amid the constant stream of new diet books.

But like so many people, I'm a product of this fad diet system. And also like so many, I never quite had the rigid discipline and self-control that was called for to stay on these diets for more than a few weeks (maybe a month, tops). The sad irony is that when I'd go back to just eating healthy, I would always gain weight. Why? Because whatever diet I had been on was not right for my body and totally unsustainable. No one wants to be on a diet. But we also don't trust ourselves without a plan. What I really needed was nonexistent. I wanted a real *lifestyle* plan, light structure around what was healthy to stay balanced, and a contingency plan for celebrating life. But most important, I wanted to feel empowered.

This is not to say that I didn't find *any* useful information in those books—I did; I found a lot. My inner geek soaked up nuggets of nutritional science, biology, anatomy, pharmacology, biochemistry—whatever I could find. And often this information made sense, especially if it was packaged or associated with a plan that helped me lose weight. But whatever the strategy—no carb, low carb, no fat, low fat, all cabbage, just juice—I'd always, *always* gain back the weight I'd lost, because I couldn't sustain it. So for all the good information and diets that delivered results, I was in constant fear that those results were just temporary. And they so often were.

I realized I needed to know even more. I wanted to see the studies supporting dietary claims. Why were there were so many contradictions? When I'd do a first round of research on the Internet, I'd find dozens of theories, contradictions, and biased studies that had gone viral, only adding to and exacerbating the misinformation and confusion out there. For instance, you might recall the study that claimed that soy can help prevent breast cancer. It was cited 347 times. What?! I worked in oncology for six years and know that breast tumors that are estrogen receptor (ER) positive will *grow* when fed estrogen. So why would we recommend soy, a product full of phytoestrogen, as a prevention strategy? Six other studies went the other way and explained soy's potential role in tumor growth. But what's cited and goes viral too often becomes the "truth," both anecdotal and otherwise.

So I decided to dig deeper than the first page of my Google search results. I used my research skills, went to the source, and read the actual studies. I mined PubMed articles and began to separate the studies that had been replicated from those that made bold, often exaggerated or even misleading claims. Gradually, I became aware of two important realities:

1. We are only at the tippy-top of the iceberg when it comes to nutritional research. In a lot of instances, studies are funded by big business, which limits and dictates what gets researched. To make matters more complicated, government agencies offer advice that is somehow always pro the industry they regulate (as with the U.S. Department of Agriculture [USDA], which is very pro-agribusiness). It comes at the expense of our health, further muddying the waters for people about what is safe to buy in our grocery stores, never mind holding back the advancement of continued education in nutrition. To say that more research is needed is a huge understatement.

2. The knowledge landscape is always in flux, constantly evolving. For instance, only a few short years ago, scientists believed mapping the human genome

would unravel the diseases plaguing our society. We were told in big, front-page headlines that genes held the answers to all our current health problems. Today, only a few short years later, scientists tell us that genes are only *one facet* of understanding our individual health signature, and they can't possibly explain or deliver the solutions we were hoping for. They pivoted to what they believe is a more comprehensive way to understand the great complexity of human health and disease states. This new understanding of how our genetic inheritance constantly interacts with the environment is called **epigenetics**.

Epigenetics is an important development to note. Any one of us might carry the biomarker for certain diseases—cancer, heart disease, or diabetes, for example—but that disease might get triggered only if a certain lifestyle (such as a stressful physical and/or emotional environment) is present. Molecules produced by our healthy gut bacteria play a very important role in either directly or indirectly affecting epigenetic processes in the body. (See Your Gut Health, page 226.) Our diet also plays a vital role in maintaining the health of the microorganisms living in and on our body (our **macrobiota**). In other words, we may be able to avoid certain diseases if we live healthier lifestyles. New research even suggests that our gut microbiota influences our glycemic responses to foods. This connection between lifestyle, microbiota, and the human genome is proof that we need to strive for clean eating, real food, and balanced meals with high nutrition built in, and not jump on gimmicky gut health fads.

MAKING SENSE OF IT ALL

The Fab Four formula is the result of my life experience and my multiyear deep dive into diet books and hard-core nutritional science. At a certain point after college, while working in oncology, I realized that my passion for understanding the science of food, the biomechanics of weight loss, and the reasons that people respond so differently to foods and diets had become my day job, even though it really wasn't. I had begun helping friends and family reverse all sorts of conditions, including food allergies, inflammation, and insulin resistance. I understood what these results meant: that balancing blood sugar and eating a nutritious lifestyle—a Fab Four lifestyle—meant that I was onto something important. And that's when, with the encouragement of my husband, I decided I would focus all my energy on helping people discover the balance and food freedom that I now enjoy.

What have I learned since then? What drives my practice to help clients hit goals and stop obsessing over food? What helps them lose weight so they can look and feel amazing, whatever that means to them? What is the key to avoiding disease and setting yourself up for personal food freedom in the long term? **Light structure based on the science of balanced blood sugar and eating to satiety.** Not a rigid, rule-filled diet.

Since I've done the research, I can cut through all the noise out there in magazines and books, online and on podcasts, and in the news. How are you supposed to have any idea what's right for you or anybody else? I take great pleasure and pride in sifting through the ocean of dense and conflicting information for my clients, to help them silence the noise and simply be able to live. I developed that same holistic, personalized approach for my clients that I did for myself.

My hundreds of personal clients vary in age, backgrounds, and walks of life. From business professionals and NFL athletes to teens, brides, and new moms; from actors and television hosts who want to look great on-camera to clients afflicted with gout, leaky gut, celiac disease, gestational diabetes, rheumatoid arthritis, high cholesterol, PCOS, diabetes, and psoriasis. Two quick success stories:

John, a forty-year-old CEO of a multimillion-dollar beauty company, was suffering from high cholesterol and a stubborn belly roll. He was what I call a "high-cholesterol pescatarian" who didn't eat red meat and relied mostly on fish and soy for his protein. But he wasn't getting enough protein or good fat. When we removed the soy-protein-bar snacks, high-carb breakfast cereal, and champagne with dinner, and replaced them with #Fab4 meals (a combination of foods based around the essential macronutrients—protein, fat, fiber, and greens) and a Fab Four Smoothie, John not only lost eight pounds but reduced his cholesterol significantly.

Bethany, a thirty-five-year-old mother of three, wanted to show her daughters good eating habits, but she also wanted to lose some weight. She was eating scrambled egg whites and tablespoons of almond butter for breakfast, but starving herself the rest of the day, so she was always hungry. She was also working out excessively and not sleeping. When we made a few simple changes to both the timing and content of her meals, she not only lost weight (ten pounds in four weeks!) but began sleeping through the night, and stopped feeling anxious and hungry all the time.

John and Bethany both learned how to make food decisions that would balance their blood sugar, and how to eat to satiety. My Fab Four formula works for all sorts of people because it's both specific and personalized. Clients learn how *their* blood sugar curve works, what triggers hunger and inflammation, and what a balanced meal really looks like. If you put protein, fat, fiber, and greens on your plate at every meal, and feel and see the results, then you are empowered to eat that way. You quickly learn the joy and relief of feeling relaxed around food. And you'll avoid those strict, zero-tolerance diet rules that make you feel confined, food obsessed, and guilty when you don't hit the mark.

My approach isn't about rules or eat-and-don't-eat lists. I help my clients understand what happens in their body when they eat certain foods, and from there figure out simple principles to guide their diet, nutrition, and lifestyle decisions. If you know why something is good for you (or not); if you know how something will optimize your body's performance (or not); and if you know how your body works (and doesn't), then the shackles come off and you find freedom. By contrast, diets tend to lock you up somewhere else: scale jail.

One of the key things I've learned is that we all have our range: our fit range and our fat range. You know that feeling of being a few pounds down, when everything is great? It *is* great. Then you relax a bit, stop being so hypervigilant, and enjoy yourself a little. Soon you indulge yourself right back into your fat range, so you run to whatever quick-fix fad diet sounds best and hop on board, hoping you can stick with it for more than seventy-two hours. These types of cycles and weight swings are a form of torture, as we watch the scale (and ourselves) with no real sense of control.

But what's really crazy is expecting our weight to be stagnant or fixed. Unfortunately, this is the underlying expectation of many diets. In reality, the body has a normal range or equilibrium, called **homeostasis**. But that's all it is: a range! It might sound clichéd, but the only constant is change—our body is always regulating our acidity and alkalinity, body temperature, and blood pH. Most of the time our cells do fine, automatically balancing our blood sugar and other contributing factors. In fact, right now millions of cells have channels and membranes that are bringing nutrients into your cells and pushing nutrients out, and a lot can change in a day.

Let's just look at fluid. You can sweat anywhere from 1.5 gallons (average) up to 4 gallons (hard work) in just one day. (For reference, 1 gallon of water weighs 8.34 pounds.) This doesn't mean you can lose 12 actual pounds in a day, but it points to how our bodies react strongly to do what we do . . . or don't do. Beyond hydration levels, our body weight is controlled by our conscious actions to stop eating when we're full, go to bed early, and get in enough movement. Knowing how to connect to this built-in ideal body weight isn't all automatic. It's highly emotional and conscious—it takes awareness of how we feel. So it would actually be surprising for us to weigh the same amount day after day.

When you live the Fab Four lifestyle, you'll stop living and dying by the scale. You'll focus on nourishing your body, trusting its signals, and looking and feeling vibrant *for yourself,* not the scale. So if the goal is not to achieve a fixed, ideal weight, what is the goal?

Balance. Scale homeostasis.

Balance isn't easy. Trust me, I've been there. I still experience an internal struggle over finding it. I want to be the life of the party, pouring the vino and making my best friends laugh. But I also want cucumber water, hot baths, HIIT (high-intensity interval training), and yoga classes. Balance is having them both, and freedom is ditching restrictive diets and using *knowledge* as your guide. When you feel out of balance, you're not yourself. If you enjoy going out with friends but tend to gain weight when you do, you can become afraid to leave the safety of home, where it's easier to control your food choices and avoid a world of options that might make you inflamed or bloated or gain weight. But what if you knew you wouldn't have to panic about going out? To know that if you plan to go wine tasting on the weekend, you can prepare accordingly and auto-correct quickly? That's the Fab Four formula.

All restrictive diets eventually implode, leaving you feeling less confident than you were when you started. Our inability to stay on plan can wreak havoc, setting off a cascade of insecurity that sends ripples into other areas of your life—relationships, work, family. How is that healthy? It's *not.* Enough dieting! (And for goodness' sake, this is not the time to snag a three-day juice cleanse. The weight loss is only temporary, and in the end you'll be left feeling irritable and full of cravings. In other words, **Do not pass go, do not collect $200, go directly to scale jail!**)

My plan encourages you to celebrate within reason, knowing you can bring yourself back into alignment. Bingeing and cleansing cycles swing you back and forth like an out-of-control pendulum, but happiness and health are attained when you find balance. But balance isn't when you stop moving and live a rigid, overly planned, supposedly perfect life. You are human. None of us is perfect. You will swing a little from time to time. We all do. Balance is found with intentional movement to eat clean, sweat often, and even enjoy a glass of wine with friends. Accept who you are, love who you are, and build a lifestyle focused on health, not some abstract idea of perfection. Punishing yourself for "failing" is unhealthy and unproductive, and breeds disappointment.

You just need light direction. And you can think of this book as the bumpers on your bowling lane.

HOW MOST DIETS STEER YOU WRONG

I didn't create my company to bash all the diets out there—they're generally well-intentioned and simply exist to help people lose weight. The good ones are based on unbiased scientific studies with significant p-values (i.e., a strong probability of outcome), explain common medical issues, and explore real success stories. But here's why they end up not working: (1) most "livable" plans work only in an antisocial vacuum; (2) they expect you to have an unemotional relationship with food; (3) they require hour upon hour of preparation in the kitchen; (4) they don't account for travel, celebrations, or *real life*; and (5) most are "all or nothing."

Many diets require you to make wholesale lifestyle changes all at once. That's a tall order for anyone, and doesn't set you up for success. Further, diets can keep you vulnerable to cravings, set you up for food obsession, and make you overthink calories. Dramatic food claims have you cutting out perfectly good food options and petrified to eat out. Many diets are so restrictive in their food choices that you begin to resent them. The doughnut you weren't going to

13

eat anyway now haunts your "do not eat" dreams. And when you go off plan, you "fail." What?! You're forced to either look for the next quick fix or start all over again tomorrow, Monday, or next month. It's the "diet mentality" and subsequent binges that keep us addicted to foods that trigger disease, because essentially you're only ever *on* or *off* plan. How is that sustainable?

Let's say you start a new plan and are 100 percent committed to never eating rice again. But what happens when eventually you want sushi? Will it be the sugar-laden white rice or the arsenic-rich brown rice? You see, I can give you a number of reasons you should have one over the other (or none), but wellness isn't the result of a binary decision. Ultimately, my recommendation would depend on what else you were eating with that meal, what you ate earlier that day, your daily workout schedule, and most importantly, what you like best. (When was the last time you asked yourself that?) Diets focus on fear and restriction, with a side of doomsday. It always reminds me of the Ellen DeGeneres stand-up bit about the obviousness of antidepressant commercials: "All the commercials on TV today are for antidepressants, for Prozac or Paxil. And they get you right away. 'Are you sad? Do you get stressed, do you have anxiety?' 'Yes, I have all those things! I'm alive!'" Do we really need to be pandered to by drug companies and reminded that life is stressful? Diet gurus do the same thing. They play on our emotions and then remind us we're destined to be a fat bag of toxins unless we comply.

One of the main ways most diets steer you wrong is by asking you to restrict or count calories, remove food groups, or weigh your food. But even if a plan doesn't specifically instruct you to track, count, and watch calories, most clients I meet with initially believe they need to reduce calories if they *really* want to lose weight. The idea of calories is so deeply ingrained in us that if we even allow ourselves to eat breakfast, we limit it to a hard-boiled egg, a nonfat latte, a protein bar, or a solo green juice. Indeed, as recently as 2015, the USDA and the Department of Health and Human Services (HHS) stated together that the best way to manage weight was to "control calorie intake" and maintain "appropriate calorie balance during each stage of life—childhood, adolescence, adulthood, pregnancy and breastfeeding, and older age." This principle has been the sometimes silent, and sometimes overt, foundation of almost every diet published over the past fifty-plus years.

But as our population has become heavier and heavier, the medical and scientific communities have begun to question this so-called medical fact. Pioneers such as doctors Robert Lustig, David Perlmutter, Mark Hyman, and David Ludwig have pushed back on this conventional wisdom and begun to size up and apply the research being done. We're starting to understand that calories don't really count—they backfire. Calorie consumption guidelines ultimately diminish our underlying trust in ourselves to make good food choices. Further, they ignore biological need, blood sugar response, and hormonal reactions. Eating those 100-calorie packs undermines and erodes an innate ability that we all possess: the body's natural drive to find its ideal weight and set point.

Diets with a light, more livable structure have grown in popularity, making it easier for people to eat successfully and ditch some drama. But there's usually a catch. For instance, "approved" sugars. We love sugar and push the limits to eat naturally occurring sugar in things like coconut flour cookies, almond meal banana bread, or simply lots of fruit. But even a "naturally occurring" sugar will affect your blood sugar, inflammation levels, and hormones.

I know the effect of certain diets and types of foods because I examine my clients' lab results firsthand. I read lab reports (blood, urine, stool, and spit) from a nutrition standpoint, looking for high glucose, cholesterol, and cortisol and other indications of inflammation, like C-reactive protein and interleukin-6. Then I help clients build individual plans to fix their issues or reach their goals with real food.

When thirty-year-old Eric came to me, he had been fighting gout for three years. His doctor had simply told him to stop eating red meat and drinking wine to lower his uric acid levels—this without even asking Eric what he was eating in the first place. (Did you know most doctors are required to take only twenty-three hours total of nutrition training during twelve years of education and preparation to practice medicine?) When we went over Eric's food habits and I checked his lab results, it was clear that the real culprit for his gout was the sour candy he ate all the time—candy laden with high-fructose corn syrup! Eric hasn't had a gout attack in the four years he's been on the Fab Four program.

Diets also reinforce people's belief that they are not in control of their bodies. If a diet comes with a "good food" list and a "bad food" list, then it's setting you up to think, *Okay, I can eat this, but not that. If I stick only to these foods* [restriction!], *I will lose weight. If I eat anything from the bad list* [shame!], *then the diet won't work.* This mental cycle fuels food obsession, which is the opposite of food freedom and is doomed to fail you eventually (not the other way around). And even if a food is on the "good" or "approved" list, this doesn't mean it will set you up for success. It might buy you a ticket on the blood sugar roller coaster.

On a biological level, a grain-free doughnut, açai bowl, and steel-cut oatmeal can all cause a disturbance or imbalance in blood sugar. Although they may contain "superfoods," those superfoods are still carbohydrates that are digested into glucose and spike your blood sugar. Your body doesn't like these aggressive spikes and works to restore blood sugar balance with insulin. Insulin is a hormone made in your pancreas that ferries glucose out of your bloodstream (thereby lowering your blood sugar) and stores it in your liver, your muscles, and finally your fat cells. As more insulin circulates in your bloodstream, more calories are stored. The problem is that as blood sugar leaves the bloodstream, you start to feel really hungry again, you reach for a snack, and then your fat burning shuts down. This doesn't mean you can never have these foods (or that they are "bad"). But knowing they'll cause a spike-crash cycle with your blood sugar will empower you to be aware of what you're eating, learn to prepare, and know what to do to break the cycle.

In short, most diets out there don't teach us how to eat enough to keep our bodies in blood sugar balance and feel sated—that is, satisfied and content so we don't feel hungry for hours. After all, isn't that the point of food?

The good news is the minute you understand blood sugar, macronutrient metabolism, and the hormonal reactions involved, you can set yourself free. You can make a choice to eat that doughnut and then know how to stop the spike-crash cycle. The science of macronutrients also explains why your perfectly planned, packed, and calorie-calculated day has you starving, cranky, and gaining weight. A focus on calories leads you down the path to weight gain, which can also cause type 2 diabetes, metabolic syndrome, and sometimes fatty liver disease.

If you overdo carbohydrate-rich foods, restrict calories, or don't eat enough of a full range of foods, you can experience large fluctuations in blood sugar. Crashes or dips happen when your pancreas overdoes it and insulin transfers too much sugar out of the bloodstream and into the cells. *Oops.* Large variations in blood sugar paired with excess insulin leave you feeling hungry, weak, shaky, light-headed, and anxious. Been there? Maybe it's because you started your day with cereal or were juicing, or maybe you just grabbed a protein bar or a nonfat latte because you were traveling and didn't have a chance. Whatever the reason, the result is you begin to crash, craving sugar and carbohydrates.

These cravings don't come out of nowhere; they're predictable. When your blood sugar starts to drop, you're hardwired to eat. Hormonal hunger happens when our blood sugar starts to drop even when it's in the normal range

BUYER BEWARE

Side note—stop paying for expensive meal delivery programs based on calories! Not only do these programs set you up to stay calorie-obsessed, but they also undermine your confidence that you have control over your body, your weight, and the foods you put in your mouth. What's worse? They solidify the habit to eat every few hours without understanding the hormonal consequences. I understand the need for convenience, but I promise, Fab Four recipes are simple, fast, and made with real, macronutrient-dense foods that will help you lose weight and make you full!

17

and can have your reaching for another snack as early as 90 minutes after your last meal. In fact, your hormones make you think of carbohydrates (which are high-glycemic) because they typically guarantee quick energy and represent the fastest way to get more glucose into your system. When your body thinks it may be starving, your brain purposefully suggests you eat foods that provide a short-term fix (*"We need candy! Sugary granola bars! Breeeeeeeeead!"*), despite the long-term health and weight consequences.

The problem with this short-term fix is that it starts the blood sugar roller coaster all over again. Ever had one of those days when you take five laps to see "what's in the fridge" over and over again? Welcome to a very addictive and frustrating loop: spike in blood sugar > surge of insulin > dip in blood sugar > insatiable carb craving > crazy addict in search of a candy bowl > and up you go again. And in the process, your body shuts down its fat-burning mode and stores more fat. This is the cycle that begins, for example, if you have carbs for breakfast, lunch, and dinner.

What does this teach us about how and why people gain weight, lose weight, and pack it on again? That when our bodies don't get the nutrition they need, they try to work around the problem with hormones, and these workarounds cause cravings, binges, more fat storage, and an insatiable hunger.

As human beings, we're driven to feel satiated. We're driven to eat food for our survival. And our bodies are designed to be healthy and function optimally when they receive a mix of essential macronutrients—the Fab Four: **fibrous and green carbohydrates** (for energy and good-bacteria proliferation), **protein** (for cell and tissue growth), and **fat** (for brain functioning, hormone production, and immune protection). When the body doesn't get sufficient amounts of these food sources, or the foods come in a form that has been modified by chemicals or is low in nutrients, the body adjusts in a number of negative ways, most of which lead to weight gain and inflammation. Without the clean, nutrient-dense forms of these macronutrients, the body can't break down food completely, so it stores it as fat and makes you feel hungry, no matter how much you eat. Ultimately, the body might turn on itself and develop diseases such as atherosclerosis, diabetes, and cancer.

You might not be worried about these medical conditions now, but this same cycle of eating foods that your body can't break down also affects how you look and feel *now*. Dry or oily skin? Stubborn muffin top? Thinning hair? Puffy or red eyes? All signs that your body might not be getting the nutrition it needs.

#FAB4 TO THE RESCUE!

We've been told by many a diet book that we should eat every three to four hours. But why? Well, on average, your blood sugar rises when you eat and starts to fall three hours later. But this advice doesn't take into account what you ate, how much you ate, the time of day, where your blood sugar started, your current blood sugar level, or your insulin and cortisol levels. And what about glucagon, the hormone that releases *stored* blood sugar? Glucagon is a fat-burning hormone that raises your blood sugar by converting glycerol in your fat cells to glucose for fuel, lowers the production of LDL ("bad cholesterol"), and lets your body release excess fluid. Why would we have such a hormone if we were never going to use it?

Digestion is work for our bodies; it takes a lot of time and energy to break down food into molecules that we can then absorb and utilize. When we eat too frequently, we're taxing our body, filling it with excess insulin, and asking it to restart a process it has not yet completed. Not only does this weigh us down in terms of energy depletion, but also in pounds. When our body cannot absorb and utilize food, it stores it as (you guessed it) fat.

But when you begin your day with a Fab Four Smoothie or #Fab4 breakfast from this book, you give yourself the opportunity to start and stay in a tight and balanced blood sugar state. Then, when you follow this with two other nutrient-rich meals, you can elongate your blood sugar curve into a normal range. The result? You don't get cravings and you lose weight! You're also re-teaching your body how to feel full and satisfied, so that between your meals you're actually burning fat and losing weight instead of impatiently waiting for your next snack.

DITCH DIETS FOREVER

One of the biggest truths I've discovered is that the body is an amazing feat of nature. It is designed to work, be healthy, and protect itself from disease and the environment. It's also driven toward satiety and to find its optimal weight. When the body is given whole, clean food sources, it will work in perfect harmony, naturally falling into homeostasis and balance. It will feel nourished and content and, as a result, arrive at the optimal weight for that individual. In this way, the body is simple.

Here's how.

2
YOU'VE GOT TO START SOMEWHERE . . .

. . . SO WHY NOT START with the knowledge that will help set you free!

What follows in this chapter is a short but immensely powerful primer on nutrition and biology that will lay down that red carpet toward your own amazing future. If you really want to be free from diets forever, you need to understand blood sugar and some basic nutritional biology. From there, it's all light structure, the #BeWellFab4, and the Fab Four Smoothie!

But first, picture this weekend scenario. You sit down at a "healthy" brunch spot with your friends. You look at the menu and want everything. It all sounds healthy . . . kale eggs Benedict, a veggie omelet, savory Paleo breakfast meats, seven-grain vegan pancakes, açai bowls with homemade granola, even gluten-free sweets. Plus, it's the weekend and you're with your friends. A fun drink sounds, well, fun. How do you decide what to eat and drink?

Let's say you went with the seven-grain vegan pancake, a side of fruit, and a mimosa. Oh, and a bite (or two—okay, three) of the giant, gluten-free sticky bun one of your girlfriends orders for the table. (Because cheers to the freakin' weekend, right?) Well, this combination of ingredients—nonfibrous carbohydrates, sugar, and minimal protein and fat—will put you on the blood sugar roller coaster. It doesn't matter if it's vegan, gluten-free, or hipster approved. You'll spike your blood sugar so high that the only place it can go after a few hours is crashing down. The result is that you'll start craving more sugar and nonfibrous carbohydrates.

Why? Because you're hardwired to eat, and your hormones tell you to eat food that will raise your blood sugar as quickly as possible. By four P.M., you may be curled up in your pajamas, watching Netflix, ready to order a pizza for an early dinner, make a bag of popcorn, or take down a bag of cookies. But the reality (and good news) is that you're not physically hungry. You're hormonally hungry and full of insulin.

Back to that delicious brunch. Let's say you went with the veggie omelet, added avocado (or heck, even bacon), and a side of spinach or salad, and went with a vodka-soda with a squeeze of lemon. This combination of ingredients—protein (egg, bacon), fat (avocado), and fibrous carbohydrates (spinach, veggies)—will make you feel full and satisfied, and you won't crave more food in two or three hours. Why? Because it won't dramatically spike your blood sugar outside a normal range, which means you won't experience a corresponding dramatic crash. Your hunger hormones stay under control. This meal will elongate your blood sugar curve (fat and fiber help to do that) and should keep you happy for four to six hours, depending on your unique body chemistry. Hey, and you had a few sips of fun, too.

These two scenarios show how your body reacts to create blood sugar, one of our primary sources of energy. In essence, your body metabolizes and absorbs food by breaking down different food groups (macronutrients) into usable forms for cells to function. This is what we think of as digestion.

For me, when I went back to where I began—understanding the basics about digestion and blood sugar—I had completed my quest: I understood how to lose weight, how to eat for wellness and maintenance, and best of all, how to stop my cravings and preoccupation with food. If you know what your body needs and what will balance and elongate—not spike and crash—your blood sugar curve, you will have the keys to the **Fab Four** kingdom and a recipe for food freedom.

BIOLOGY 101

If you were to break your body into its components, it would look something like this: 64 percent water, 19 percent protein (muscles), 16 percent fat, 4 percent minerals (such as the calcium and phosphorus in your bones and the iron in your blood), and 1 percent carbohydrates (mostly glucose in your bloodstream or glycogen—stored glucose—in your liver or muscles). Your body is constantly breaking down old, oxidized cells and synthesizing new ones. In fact, in your lifetime, you will synthesize somewhere between 550 and 950 pounds of protein! So yes, you really are reinventing yourself daily.

But how, and with what? The "how" is two metabolic processes, known as **catabolism** (to break down and release energy) and **anabolism** (to build and consume energy). And the "what" is what you eat—the nutrients in the food and liquids you consume. There are macronutrients (carbohydrates, protein, and fat), micronutrients (vitamins and minerals), phytonutrients (antioxidants), and water. Let's start with the macronutrients.

The majority of your food is made up of macronutrients. Very few foods contain just one macronutrient—meat is made up of both protein and fat; vegetables are fiber-rich carbohydrates that can also contain protein; even chia seeds contain protein, fat, and fiber. But more often than not, if a food contains a single macronutrient, it has been extracted. For example, coconut oil, avocado oil, and olive oil are all 100 percent fat, but the whole food (the avocado, coconut, or olive) contains a mixture of carbohydrates, proteins, water, and other micro- or phytonutrients. (For the sake of simplicity, however, I will categorize foods by their predominant macronutrient.)

The three macronutrients—carbohydrates, protein, and fat—have different nutritional functions, and each is used and breaks down differently in your metabolic processes.

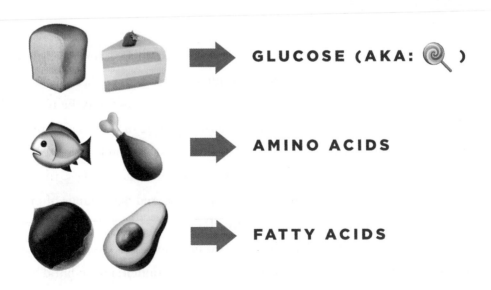

- **CARBOHYDRATES** break down into **glucose** (or blood sugar), a type of sugar that gives our cells energy. There are two general types of carbohydrates, both of which are plant-based: (1) simple carbohydrates, which are easily broken down into glucose; and (2) complex carbohydrates, which are "wrapped" in fiber and more difficult to break down. Simple carbohydrates come in many different forms, but think *sugar* when you think *simple*: table sugar, corn syrup, honey, jams and jellies, soda, and candy. Some of these simple sugars can be found in raw sugarcane, honey, and even fruit, but many are processed one way or another. (Of note, the sugar fructose is metabolized differently, which we'll discuss in a little bit.) Complex carbohydrates come in a much wider variety of foods: green vegetables; fruit; whole grains (including oatmeal, pasta, and whole-grain breads); rice, wheat; seeds and nuts; starchy vegetables such as potatoes, corn, and squash; and beans, lentils, and peas (also known as legumes).

- **PROTEINS** break down into **amino acids**, which enable our muscles and other tissues to build and stay strong. However, our bodies can produce only thirteen out of the twenty-two amino acids that make up proteins. The nine amino acids our bodies can't manufacture are known as "essential," and we need to get them from plant- or animal-based sources. For instance, fish, beef, pork, chicken, and eggs are all examples of complete animal-based proteins. Complete plant-based proteins include quinoa, buckwheat (not a grain!), and chickpeas. And here's that vegetarian caveat: plant proteins in their natural form are mostly carbohydrates. To get 8 grams of protein from quinoa, you need to process roughly 40 grams of carbohydrates. To get 20 grams of protein from chickpeas, you need to process roughly 60 grams of carbohydrates. Spoiler alert: That affects your blood sugar! Later, in chapter 6, I will help you strategize about how to make sure you have the right amount of protein for you.

- **FATS** break down into various types of **fatty acids**, which enable hormone production and cell development and growth. Our main sources of "good" fats are avocados, fatty fish (such as salmon, trout, mackerel, sardines, and herring), olive oil, coconut and coconut oil, nuts, and chia seeds, not to mention dark chocolate! Soon we'll dive a little deeper into fats, including the different types, their sources, and how the body and brain use them. We'll also discuss the essential fatty acids, omega-3 and omega-6. You'll see how important fat is to feeling good and **being well!**

On top of these macronutrients, your body also needs micronutrients (vitamins and minerals) and phytonutrients (antioxidants). Our bodies process these from the macronutrients we eat. But if the carbohydrates, proteins, and fats we're eating are not of high quality (they're processed, industrially raised, overcooked, or sullied by chemicals), then it's important to rely on supplements to make sure your brain and body get sufficient amounts (this is discussed in detail in chapter 10).

Water is also vital to our very survival and ensures the proper balance of fluid, both inside and outside our cells. It assists with nervous system, temperature regulation, muscle functioning, nutrient transport, and proper excretion of wastes from the body to avoid toxicity. Not listening? Dehydration will age you!

So how is all this nutrient stuff going to help you ditch diets forever? When you eat clean, nutrient-dense forms of macronutrients (the Fab Four), you will keep your blood sugar in balance and feel sated, naturally turning off your "hunger" hormones and stopping the spike-crash-crave cycle before it starts.

Remember that USDA Food Pyramid we've been seeing for the past umpteen years? Not only is it inaccurate in terms of the best sources of our macronutrients, but its arrangement is asking for diabetes. The new USDA MyPlate attempts to help us map out our meals, but where's the fat? Why are we still recommending grains and dairy at every single meal? Even the new Healthy Eating Plate from Harvard suggests three carbohydrates in one sitting (in other words, a "triple spike"), recommending fruit, grains, and dairy at every meal, and again leaving out fat.

These rankings don't get the macronutrients quite right. They overprescribe the wrong forms of carbohydrates and underprescribe the good types of fats. My formula—the Fab Four—is different (and effective) because it looks at macronutrients from the perspective of balancing your blood sugar and decreasing inflammation.

FOOD GUIDE PYRAMID
A GUIDE TO DAILY FOOD CHOICES

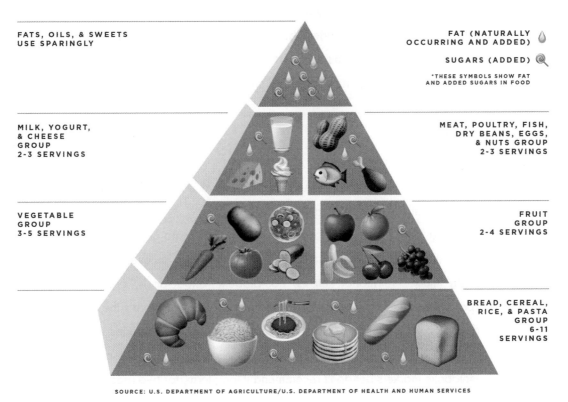

FATS, OILS, & SWEETS
USE SPARINGLY

FAT (NATURALLY
OCCURRING AND ADDED)

SUGARS (ADDED)

*THESE SYMBOLS SHOW FAT
AND ADDED SUGARS IN FOOD

MILK, YOGURT,
& CHEESE
GROUP
2-3 SERVINGS

MEAT, POULTRY, FISH,
DRY BEANS, EGGS,
& NUTS GROUP
2-3 SERVINGS

VEGETABLE
GROUP
3-5 SERVINGS

FRUIT
GROUP
2-4 SERVINGS

BREAD, CEREAL,
RICE, & PASTA
GROUP
6-11
SERVINGS

SOURCE: U.S. DEPARTMENT OF AGRICULTURE/U.S. DEPARTMENT OF HEALTH AND HUMAN SERVICES

This is how I'd like you to think of food groups and the essential nutrients we need to eat:

Most nutritionists and doctors will very quickly tell you that carbohydrates are the primary source of fuel for the human body, particularly for neurologic functions and physical exercise. But let's be clear—there isn't an "essential" carbohydrate. Think of it this way: In terms of fuel, your body is like a Toyota Prius, which can run on gasoline or battery power. Likewise, your body can run on glucose produced from the carbohydrates you eat or fat-based fuel called **ketones**. Your body can even produce glucose from noncarbohydrate sources through a process called gluconeogenesis. So carbohydrates are not your body's only source of energy. Further, my approach shifts away from low-nutrient forms of carbohydrates such as grains, pasta, bread, and potatoes and toward more nutrient-rich forms, such as colorful nonstarchy vegetables, low-glycemic fruits, beans, nuts, and seeds. These complex carbohydrate sources are the fiber and greens in the #Fab4 and will provide your body with the energy it needs without massively spiking your blood sugar.

KETOSIS

You might have heard of nutritional ketosis, a state where your body burns only fat for energy, aka battery power mode. Nutritional ketosis has attracted a lot of interest and for good reason—it's being used therapeutically to lower epileptic seizures, starve cancer, and improve recovery from traumatic brain injury. Nutritional ketosis, not diabetic ketoacidosis, provides muscle-sparing fat loss and is showing to be neuroprotective. What's the catch? It's a difficult state to maintain without a strict diet, exogenous ketones, and the constant monitoring of blood or urine. In my practice, I use it periodically to improve metabolic markers but don't recommend it long-term, for two reasons: (1) carbohydrates help produce the mucus that protects our intestines and promotes gut health; (2) colorful carbohydrate foods (like beets, carrots, and squash) contain vitamins, minerals, and phytonutrients—nutrients I don't want my clients avoiding to stay in ketosis.

Now let's turn to fats, an important macronutrient for the body. They break down into various types of fatty acids, which enable hormone production and cell development and growth, and also are critical for blood sugar balance. Yet they're often not emphasized enough.

Fats come in three basic forms: triglycerides, phospholipids, and sterols. We rely most on triglycerides. Some triglycerides are good and necessary (they make up 60 percent of our brain and protect our heart), but others can interfere with our health by causing inflammation, clogged arteries, and high blood pressure. On the "good" side, there are **monounsaturated** fats from olive oil, avocados, and nuts; long-chain **polyunsaturated omega-3** fats from algae and fish and other seafood; and **saturated fats** from coconut, red palm oil, and pasture-raised animals and eggs. As for the "bad" fats, these are **trans-unsaturated** fats (trans fats) and man-made industrial seed oils (such as canola, sunflower, safflower, cottonseed, grapeseed, corn, soybean, or vegetable oil). These processed oils contain excessive amounts of omega-6, which can cause inflammation. (Tip: If a label reads "partially hydrogenated," steer clear!)

The body is capable of producing all the fatty acids it needs except for two. They're "essential" because we need to get them from our food. The first is **linoleic acid** (LA), an inflammatory omega-6. Now, just because LA is inflammatory doesn't mean it's bad. For instance, when you bump your knee and it swells, that's LA supporting the inflammatory phase of wound healing, sending nutrients and blood flow to the area. So don't believe the hype that omega-6 from organic whole foods like eggs, nuts, seeds, and grass-finished meats are an issue. Those foods are great sources of essential omega-6 fats that provide B vitamins like choline and folate, tocopherols, polyphenols, magnesium, fiber, and amino acids.

The second essential fatty acid is **alpha-linolenic acid** (ALA), an anti-inflammatory omega-3. At the risk of getting a little too technical, our body uses ALA to make two long-chain omega-3 fatty acids—**eicosapentanaenoic acid** (EPA) and **docosahexaenoic acid** (DHA). These are the "fish oil" fats, and you can get what you need from algae or the seafood that eats algae, like fish and shellfish. But our body isn't very good at producing EPA and DHA. In fact, only 5 percent of ALA gets converted to EPA, and less than 1 percent of ALA is converted to DHA. But though we get "omega-3" ALA from flax, chia, and walnuts, it's not the only kind your body needs or one that can be efficiently synthesized into EPA or DHA. The good news is that chickens are great at synthesizing ALA and converting it into EPA and DHA. So you can opt for pasture-raised chickens and eggs, which contain five times as much omega-3 as conventional eggs.

I consider EPA and DHA "essential" as well. Why? First, the anti-inflammatory benefits of omega-3 fats, such as reduction in heart disease and "bad" triglycerides, improved cognitive function and fetal development, improved immunological response, and lower levels of depression, are all linked to EPA and DHA. Second, the human body needs about a 1:1 ratio of omega-6 to omega-3 to perform optimally and stay balanced. However, most Americans have an inflammatory ratio of about 15:1 (!) with 20 percent having no detectable level of omega-3. EPA and DHA are omega-3s that can help improve the ratio.

Before you douse yourself in fish oil, let's take a minute to understand why our ratios are so high. Have you ever seen sunflower, safflower, cottonseed, grapeseed, corn, or soybean oils on an ingredient label? These oils seem to be in everything and are almost exclusively omega-6, and not the good kind. Industrial seed oils are often oxidized because of the chemical processes used to extract them or heated above their smoke point. When the body gets too much of these unhealthy seed oils or hydrogenated oils (trans fats), our ratios become unbalanced, and this results in chronic inflammation that can lead to disease.

The bottom line is that most of us don't get enough of the "good" fats that give us the building blocks for hormone production. Why not? Because most people believe erroneously that dietary fat makes you fat. Not true! The majority of fat being stored in your body starts as a carbohydrate. Which leads us back to (you guessed it) blood sugar.

So let's take a closer look at how your body breaks down carbohydrates.

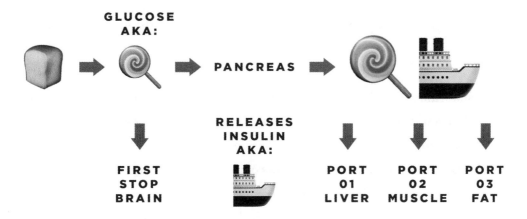

TRACKING CARBOHYDRATES

As with any other food, the process begins in your mouth and stomach, where enzymes and hydrochloric acid go to work. Carbohydrates are metabolized (broken down) into glucose, or blood sugar. As seen in the diagram above, glucose can be used by the brain without the help of insulin. However, all the remaining glucose must be managed by the hormone insulin, which is produced by your pancreas. Insulin is the storage hormone that allows glucose to move from the bloodstream into your cells. It's up to insulin to keep an appropriate amount of glucose circulating in your bloodstream (the so-called normal range of blood sugar is between 70mg/ml and 120mg/ml) and deliver appropriate amounts to your cells for energy.

Imagine insulin as a cargo ship with customs paperwork that is sent out by the pancreas to pick up glucose from your bloodstream and deliver it to a specific port of call. The three ports of call for glucose are the liver cells, muscle cells, and fat cells. Depending on the port, the pancreas might be required to submit more or less paperwork (more or less insulin) to enter. Further, when the insulin gets to a port, it signals for the cell to accept the glucose it's transporting.

1. Small amounts of insulin are used by the *liver* to process and store glucose as glycogen. The liver can store between 250 and 500 calories of glucose before it fills up.

2. Your *muscles* require large amounts of insulin to process and store glucose, but they can store between 800 and 2,000 calories (in your body as a whole) before they fill up. Once glucose "de-boards" and stores as glycogen, the only way to make room for more in your muscles is for you to move or work out. In other words, you gotta burn it! If you are moving, you are constantly making room for visitors and keeping "slips" at the port open for the next insulin-glucose "shipment." This is called keeping your insulin sensitivity strong, and explains why athletes and very active people can typically eat more carbohydrates—their muscles are constantly burning glucose and making room for more to be stored as energy in their muscle cells. When you aren't moving or working out, your muscles doesn't have any slips open. Your insulin sensitivity weakens and it will take *more* insulin just to get even

a fraction more glucose into any open slips. Further, when insulin levels are continually high in response to a diet that is made up of a high proportion of starchy and simple carbohydrates, muscle cells can become resistant to the "signal" insulin sends for them to accept glucose, which is known as **insulin resistance**. If your cells resist the signal, the glucose doesn't get unloaded and stays in your bloodstream, resulting in high blood sugar levels.

3. Finally, whatever excess glucose is not used by the brain, liver, and muscles is converted into free fatty acids and then stored in *fat cells* as triglycerides. You can see the issue here—when glucose stops being fuel, it starts being converted into fat.

Despite what you constantly read in articles and diet books, managing blood sugar is *not* achieved by eating five or six small meals a day. Blood sugar balance is managed with proper nutrition; various hormones, including adrenal and thyroid hormones; and stress management. As you will come to learn, the Fab Four provide your body with the right nutrition to stay balanced, instead of signaling your adrenals or thyroid gland to step in and help.

I promised to talk about fructose, a carbohydrate found in fruit and honey. Fructose is metabolized differently from other carbohydrates and turns into fat more quickly. Broken down 100 percent in the liver, fructose becomes glycerol (a sugar alcohol), which then converts free fatty acids into fat. (For reference, only 80 percent of alcohol and 20 percent of glucose is metabolized in the liver.)

So what does this mean for you? Basically, the more fructose you consume, the more fat you store. In addition, as part of the metabolic process, fructose replaces liver glycogen (which serves as energy storage). When you juice, you're *excessively* replacing liver glycogen, building up way more fructose than you need. All the excess will be stored as (you guessed it) fat.

The metabolism of fructose also results in waste products and toxins that can drive up blood pressure and lead to conditions such gout. What's more, fructose undergoes a chemical reaction that can result in liver inflammation, just like alcohol. Long-term excess fructose consumption causes high cholesterol, insulin resistance, and fat buildup in the liver and abdomen (called lipogenesis) that has been linked to metabolic syndrome and obesity.

So do I eat fruit? Yes, but I keep it to just a single serving daily. It's not an every-meal thing. (When we get to chapters 6 and 8, you'll get more info on how and when to enjoy fruit . . . and wine!)

With this understanding of how carbohydrates are metabolized, you can see why the forms of carbohydrates you eat are so important for blood sugar balance.

BLOOD SUGAR IMBALANCE

Next, let's review the types of blood sugar imbalance.

HYPERGLYCEMIA (high blood sugar) can be caused by a few different things. One is excess carbohydrates. Another is an inability to properly store blood sugar and respond to the "signal" insulin sends to muscle cells to accept glucose, which is called **insulin resistance**. In turn, insulin resistance is a metabolic risk factor for **metabolic syndrome,** or chronic (long-term and constantly recurring) hyperglycemia. Further, the stress hormone cortisol can also contribute to hyperglycemia. Elevated cortisol levels can cause an increase in blood sugar by releasing stored protein from muscles and converting it into blood sugar in the liver (gluconeogenesis). Cortisol also inhibits insulin production, which can prevent glucose from being available for immediate use. Cortisol isn't released just because of stress at work or in our personal lives. It's also produced in high amounts when our bodies are under different forms of biological stress, such as inflammation, infection, allergies, and poor sleep. All of these physical conditions can contribute to elevated cortisol and a hyperglycemic state.

HYPOGLYCEMIA (OR REACTIVE HYPOGLYCEMIA) is low blood sugar, defined as blood sugar that drops below fasting levels within four hours of eating. Reactive hypoglycemia can be caused by a number of factors, including excess insulin, insufficient response from glucagon (the hormone that releases stored sugar), insufficient cortisol response, or low thyroid function. Thyroid hormones are responsible for the output of insulin by the pancreas in response to blood sugar, the absorption of glucose by cells (GLUT 4), and clearance of insulin from the blood.

DYSGLYCEMIA is an abnormal roller-coaster ride of both high and low blood sugar, characterized by steep spikes of high blood sugar followed by reactive crashes into low blood sugar. It can be caused by any of the mechanisms cited above.

Okay, so that's the technical jargon. How will you actually *feel* when your blood sugar is imbalanced? Like you're on a roller coaster. When you have too much glucose in your bloodstream, you will feel sleepy, store excess sugar as *new* fat, and even crave sugar right after a meal. In fact, recent data is showing that the minute you start to crash, you begin to feel hungry. When you have too little glucose in your system, you feel starved, weak, shaky, light-headed, and anxious. If your meals are not balanced with the right amounts of protein, fat, fiber, and greens, you're setting yourself up to take a ride. But if you're eating clean proteins and good fats alongside fiber-rich carbohydrates, then you're more likely to keep yourself in a good blood sugar range. Your body will release less insulin, you'll avoid drastic glucose responses, and you'll feel in balance.

Let's take a closer look at the ups and downs with the help of a chart.

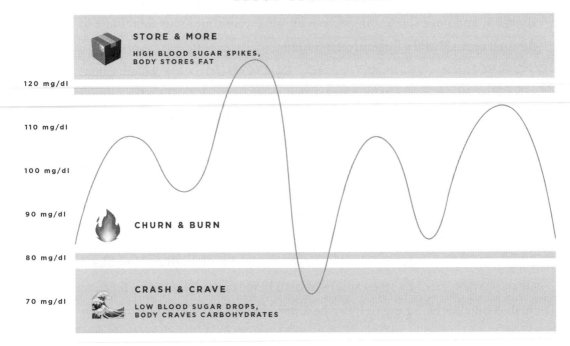

BLOOD SUGAR CHART

STORE & MORE
HIGH BLOOD SUGAR SPIKES,
BODY STORES FAT

120 mg/dl

110 mg/dl

100 mg/dl

90 mg/dl

CHURN & BURN

80 mg/dl

CRASH & CRAVE
LOW BLOOD SUGAR DROPS,
BODY CRAVES CARBOHYDRATES

70 mg/dl

THE UPS AND DOWNS OF BLOOD SUGAR

As you can see, if you start your day with a high-carbohydrate meal (such as cereal, toast, pancakes, a fruit-heavy smoothie, or even oatmeal), you set off a crazy up-and-down blood sugar cycle for the rest of the day. Your blood sugar will spike above normal and then crash, sometimes well below 80mg/dl. Dips and crashes come with strong, difficult-to-control cravings for more carbohydrates. Remember, you're hardwired to eat, and your hormones will make you seek out carbohydrates because they're the fastest way to get more glucose into your system. You'll be hormonally inclined to reach for a cookie, piece of chocolate, energy bar, or giant latte. In turn, your blood sugar will spike again, maybe even way over normal, to 125, 140, or even as high as 180mg/dl, and here we go again.

This is what happens in the bodies of most people who don't balance their meals from a macronutrient level: they become slaves to their blood sugar. Eating meals balanced with the Fab Four elongates your curve and keeps blood sugar in a normal range. It sets you free.

Okay, so let's say you don't go quite so heavy with the carbohydrates first thing in the morning. When a lot of my clients first come to me, they describe their first meal of the day as something like a nonfat latte and a KIND bar. But this breakfast lacks adequate protein, fat, and fiber to keep your blood sugar stable for four to six hours until lunch. You'll experience spikes from the lactose (sugar) in the nonfat milk and the honey and glucose syrup (sugar and sugar) in the KIND bar. But then it's 10:45 A.M., maybe only 10:30, and you start to feel hungry. Real hungry. You might reach for a snack—an apple, vanilla yogurt, even another protein bar (sugar, sugar, sugar). Or you might pour a coffee, hunker down in a deprivation mind-set, and try to hold out until lunch. In the meantime, your brain is screaming for carbohydrates. In either case, when lunch finally rolls around, your body will want to binge, either on a carb-laden meal or simply by overeating. *Coming soon: That post-lunch, could-fall-asleep-at-your-desk food coma!* Willpower lasts only so long. Your biology will always win, so you will always be a slave to your blood sugar unless you learn to manage and control it. Excessive blood sugar spikes make us sleepy, and then subsequent crashes make us crave. There's no way to sustain a pattern like this, nor would you want to. Balanced eating is everything. Balance sets you free.

Here's another thing about the blood sugar curve: See how the up-and-down cycle is happening on average about every three hours? When you eat nonfibrous, carbohydrate-rich meals without enough protein, fat, and fiber, your blood sugar spikes and you get hungry sooner and faster, perhaps in even as little as two hours, in response to your inevitable blood sugar dip. Again, how many diets do you know that recommend eating every three hours? (If you don't know, it's a lot. And it's not good for you.) These diets are simply following and reacting to this spike-crash-crave cycle, which they often cause to begin with. They recommend frequent eating because they have to. They have to answer an earlier call for more blood sugar because the foods they prescribe are not optimally balanced on the macronutrient level. I've tried these diets and usually I feel out of sorts in one form or another all day—either my blood sugar is too low, too high, or ping-ponging back and forth.

My Fab Four approach doesn't just follow and react. It anticipates, manages, and elongates your blood sugar curve. It tightens your fluctuations, sustains meals in your body, minimizes excess insulin, allows the hormone glucagon to do its job (release stored blood sugar), and naturally turns off your "hunger" hormones. Look, having glucose in your body isn't all bad. The glucose stored in your liver and muscles (glycogen) is fuel for your brain, organs, and muscles. But your need for glucose has everything to do with your activity levels. The problem is relying on carbohydrates as your main source of food. They will trigger the spike-crash-crave cycle, especially if you sit most of the day and don't work out regularly.

Think back to the brunch scenario at the beginning of this chapter. If you went for the vegan pancake, side of fruit, mimosa, and bite(s) of sticky bun, you would've been starting a metabolic process with virtually all carbohydrates, which we've seen are easily broken down into glucose. The result: The spike-crash-crave chart. If, however, you opted for the omelet with avocado (and bacon), side of spinach or salad, and vodka-soda, your blood sugar curve would look more like the chart on the next page.

When you start the day in balance, you are much more likely to stay in balance. Your blood sugar will "float" gently between 70mg/dl and 120mg/dl, without triggering cravings or out-of-control hunger. This is the gentle roll that keeps you feeling energetic but not frenetic, calm but not sedated. This is that sweet spot of being active and alert but not anxious.

BLOOD SUGAR CHART

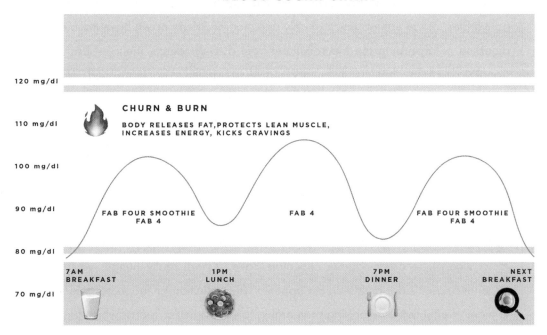

HUNGER VS. APPETITE

We're driven to eat by hunger, a physiological impulse hardwired into our brains and bodies. Hunger is regulated in the brain by the hypothalamus, which signals when the body is satiated (satisfied or full) and when it needs more food to reach that state. When we consume foods that are a healthy balance of the #BeWellFab4, our brains tell our bodies that we are sated, and we stop eating. Our bodies then begin the multi-hour process of digestion and absorption. If these food sources are clean and nutrient dense, without added ingredients that the body doesn't need, our bodies naturally use up the energy supplied by the food through our daily physical and mental activities and sleep.

However, if we consume addictive foods that are high in sugar or simple car-bohydrates, or we eat too much of only one macronutrient, or we have trouble digesting or absorbing the macronutrient from a food source, then our brain signals to our body that it is still hungry and we are driven to eat more food. We end up eating more food than our bodies and brains need.

This is the point at which most diets decide to fix the problem: they try to convince people that if they restrict or cut down on the number of calories, then they won't put their bodies in the position of storing unneeded calories. But the trouble is, simply cutting calories doesn't stop the brain from telling the body that it's hungry, which is why diets always make us feel hungry.

If you've just finished a three-course meal and find yourself still "hungry" for a slice of decadent, gooey chocolate cake, it's not really hunger you're experiencing—it's dopamine-driven appetite. The definition of "appetite" refers to more of an emotional longing or yearning to eat particular foods, which trig-gers the release of this "reward" hormone in the brain. Appetite can be aroused when environmental cues or habits stimulate our senses and make us feel happy. Think of your appetite as a psychological mechanism that drives you to seek pleasurable experiences, eating being one of them. It's very common for people to experience appetite even when they are not at all physically hungry.

We've all been through sad, stressful, emotional moments when junk or com-fort food makes us feel better. We've also been through times of joy, relaxation, and celebration when we treat ourselves. Either way, it's not the end of the world and no reason to beat yourself up with guilt, anxiety, or self-shame. You can easily smooth out any spikes in your blood sugar curve with the very next Fab Four meal.

EXCESS INSULIN

Remember when I mentioned that insulin acts like a cargo ship? It picks up glucose (blood sugar) and transfers it from your bloodstream and into your cells so that your nervous system, muscles, and other tissues and organs can use it for proper functioning. Once the insulin has done its job, it lingers in your bloodstream for six to eight hours. In the meantime, it stops the body's fat-burning process (it's a storage hormone, after all). If you eat unbalanced meals with processed foods, your blood sugar quickly rises and falls within three hours, leaving your blood low in sugar and still full of insulin. You crave and are driven to eat more carbohydrates, releasing even more insulin. This cycle of nonstop eating is known as the insulin trap, in which your body is driven to eat constantly and thus constantly produce insulin. It can also result in insulin resistance, a precursor to metabolic syndrome (chronic high blood sugar).

EXCESS INSULIN CAN CAUSE A HOST OF ISSUES, INCLUDING:

1. Increased inflammation, insulin resistance, and metabolic syndrome.
2. Increased androgens, increased testosterone in women, and increased estrogen in men (linked to PCOS, infertility, thinning hair, and acne).
3. Decreased liver detoxification and increased oxidative stress.
4. Higher blood pressure and cholesterol levels.
5. Increased fat.

The Fab Four help get you out of the trap. The foods on my program limit free-floating insulin in the first place by lowering the strength and number of blood sugar spikes (it shifts the carbohydrate focus, which means less glucose). And because the Fab Four are designed to elongate your blood sugar curve (through other macronutrients), they do so without you feeling hungry.

If, instead of processed pizza, you enjoyed roasted chicken lettuce wraps with pesto slaw and avocado, your insulin spike would be moderate and your meal would keep you satisfied for between four to six hours, depending on your unique body chemistry. Your blood sugar curve would be more of a gentle roll and less of a crashing-overhead wave. When your insulin and blood sugar curve track each other and decrease together, your glycogen and adrenal hormones can bring blood sugar back up gently, instead of being thrown into overdrive.

HORMONES THAT HELP BRING BLOOD SUGAR UP

When your blood sugar is low (below the normal range), your pancreas releases another hormone called glucagon. Glucagon acts in an opposite way to insulin: it causes the liver to convert its stored glycogen back into glucose. The glucose then reenters your bloodstream and is transported to cells for energy. Glucagon also helps break down proteins into their usable form of amino acids, which also helps to produce glucose. This is one of the reasons we don't solely need carbohydrates for glucose production. Our body has alternative ways to release and manufacture the necessary glucose.

MUSCLE WASTING

Opposed to that popular belief, this doesn't mean to prevent muscle wasting (or protein breakdown) you should eat every three hours. That theory was proven wrong by Brad Pilon years ago; muscle responds to use, stress, and challenge, not meal timing. In fact, studies have gone as low as 800 calories (80 grams of protein) per day for several weeks without a change in muscle size. Brad uses the example of wearing a cast—take off the cast and the muscle has wasted away, yet the opposite arm is still strong and the body was fed only one way. Takeaway: Use it and you won't lose it.

Hormone	Role	When things go wrong	What to do about it	How Fab Four supports
Insulin ("Storage" Hormone)	Secreted by the pancreas to allow your cells to take in glucose (blood sugar) for energy or storage. Prevents fat cells from being broken down.	Hyperinsulinemia (chronically elevated insulin), insulin resistance, metabolic syndrome, and increased hunger and cravings.	Reduce carbs to reduce chronic/ excess insulin secretion. Reduce fructose, known to increase insulin levels and linked to insulin resistance. Exercise to burn glycogen stores and increase insulin sensitivity in skeletal muscles.	Fat: Omega-3 found in fish can help lower fasting insulin levels. Greens: Magnesium found in leafy greens can improve insulin sensitivity.
Leptin ("Satiety" Hormone)	Produced by fat cells, this hormone notifies the hypothalamus (brain) that there is enough fat in storage and prevents overeating.	Leptin resistance: When impaired signaling doesn't trigger the brain to calm hunger hormones; malfunction is linked to obesity, chronically elevated insulin, and inflammation.	Avoid inflammatory foods: seed oils. Sleep: Sleep deprivation is linked to drops in leptin levels. Exercise increases leptin sensitivity.	Focus on Anti-inflammatory Fab Four (see grocery list on page 180*). Fat: Focus on omega-3 fatty acids.
Ghrelin ("Hunger" or "Gorilla" Hormone—keep eating until physically full!)	Released when the stomach is empty and stops when the stomach is stretched. Ghrelin is highest before eating and lowest an hour after eating.	Studies in obese patients show circulating ghrelin doesn't decrease and for that reason the brain doesn't receive the signal to stop eating.	Avoid white carbohydrates, sugar, and especially sugary drinks, which increase hunger without stretching the stomach lining.	Protein: Eat protein at every meal, especially breakfast, to promote satiety. Fiber: Eat foods that have mass to physically stretch the stomach lining.

Hormone	Role	When things go wrong	What to do about it	How Fab Four supports
Glucagon-Like-Peptide-1 (GLP-1) ("Full" Hormone)	Produced and released when food enters the intestines, to tell our brain we are full.	Chronic inflammation reduces GLP-1 production, which negatively affects satiety signaling.	Avoid inflammatory foods (see Oils, page 193*). Take probiotics (see page 228*).	Protein: High-protein meals increase GLP-1 production. Greens: Leafy green vegetables increase GLP-1 levels. Eat a diet of anti-inflammatory Fab Four foods (see grocery list on page 180*).
Cholecystokinin (CCK) ("Satiety" Hormone)	Produced by cells in the gastrointestinal tract and nervous system. CCK is released by the duodenum to activate the contraction of the gallbladder; secretion of gastric and pancreatic acid; slows gastric emptying; and suppresses energy metabolism.	Irritable bowel syndrome (IBS) can cause an overproduction of CCK.	A diet high in leafy greens delivers fiber and thylakoids (aka: membrane-bound compartment inside chloroplasts that contains the pigments and enzymes responsible for carrying out photosynthesis) that can double the production of CCK.	Protein: Initial studies suggest the direct interaction of CCK and dietary protein contributes to satiety response. Fat: Triggers release of CCK. Fiber: Can double CCK production!
Peptide YY (PYY) ("Control" Hormone)	Control hormone in the gastrointestinal tract that reduces appetite.	Insulin resistance and chronically elevated blood sugar impairs production of PYY.	Balanced blood sugar increases PYY response and production.	Protein: PYY concentrations increase after a protein-based meal. Fiber: Increases PYY production.

Hormone	Role	When things go wrong	What to do about it	How Fab Four supports
Neuropeptide Y (NPY) ("Stimulate" Hormone)	Hormone produced in the brain and nervous system that "stimulates" appetite for carbohydrates.	Stress induces the production of NPY that leads to appetite stimulation and overeating. Fasting and food deprivation can stimulate this hormone.	Eat complete meals regularly. Fast intermittently and with caution.	Protein: Lack of protein increases the release of NPY.
Cortisol ("Stress" Hormone)	Produced by the adrenals when the body senses stress.	Chronically elevated levels of cortisol can lead to overeating and weight gain. High levels of cortisol are linked to belly fat in women.	Manage stress levels through meditation, movement, and good sleep. Talk to loved ones and ask for help when needed.	Eat three balanced meals composed of protein, fat, fiber, and greens daily.
Dopamine ("Reward" Hormone)	Released when we eat food. This is the same hormone that is released with any form of addiction, like smoking.	Eating processed food, carbohydrates, and sugar causes a large surge in dopamine. Continuously eating these foods causes the brain to down-regulate dopamine receptors in the brain, so we need to eat more and more to get the same fix.	Eat processed foods, carbohydrates, and sugar sparingly to discourage addiction, cravings, and overeating. Eat Fab Four and always start your day with a Fab Four breakfast or protein-rich Fab Four Smoothie.	Protein: Stimulates dopamine and starts your day balanced instead of with increasing cravings throughout the day. Food addict? Make that a Cocoa Fab Four Smoothie, which increases stimulation of dopamine and balances mood swings.

At the same time, other hormones are working to increase blood sugar, including epinephrine, norepinephrine, cortisol, and growth hormone. Epinephrine and norepinephrine are secreted by the adrenal glands and nerve endings when blood sugar is low, acting on the glycogen stored in liver. This is why we get a surge of energy when we are in fight-or-flight mode. Our adrenals also secrete cortisol and growth hormone. Together, they stimulate glucose production from glycogen so muscles and other organs turn to our stored fat to use for energy.

Control of blood sugar through hormones is a healthy and normal response in the body. What isn't normal is the steep up-and-down roller coaster that comes from eating foods that quickly spike blood sugar five to six times a day, make you feel out of control, and leave you full of insulin. This cycle throws your hormones into overdrive and stresses those systems.

HOW THE FAB FOUR HELP REGULATE HORMONES

Okay, class is almost over, I promise! But before the bell rings, I want to share an important, science-based reason why I created the Fab Four.

Have you ever been on a diet and literally *fighting yourself* not to eat because you're so hungry? It's miserable! We don't do that on my program. One of the most empowering, liberating things about the Fab Four is that together they naturally balance your various hunger-related hormones. And not just for an hour. In the chart on pages 43–45, I've summarized how the Fab Four specifically help to regulate your body's hunger-related hormones.

This is a condensed, high-level summary of the very intricate way the body strives to keep itself fed and balanced, whether it is given food or not. Normally, these hormones work harmoniously, balance one another, and maintain blood sugar balance, so we never feel too hungry or eat more than is necessary for proper functioning. However, many of today's foods (even the "healthy" ones) can upset this delicate balance of hormones and disrupt overall blood sugar balance. When your hormones are out of whack, you'll feel out of whack, too!

In short, we feel best when our blood sugar and hunger-related hormones are balanced—not too high, not too low, not bonking back and forth in between, and certainly not screaming at us to eat! My approach enables you to eat in this way, so that your body hums like a Tesla. By eating a healthy combination of protein, fat, fiber, and greens, you can naturally stabilize blood sugar, burn some fat, and enjoy having consistent energy throughout the day.

Class dismissed!

3
MAKING BLOOD SUGAR BALANCE WORK FOR YOU

I'VE HAD THE GOOD fortune to counsel and coach a lot of different kinds of people. They reach out to me for one of two broad reasons: because something is ailing or bothering them, or because they have a specific goal or lifestyle they want to achieve. Their issues, symptoms, conditions, and challenges cover a very wide swath, but in my experience, many of these problems relate back to blood sugar imbalance, which has a domino effect through the whole body. We've talked about the hormonal imbalances that result in cravings, overeating, and weight gain, but beyond that, blood sugar imbalance will affect your overall health and wellness and put you at risk for serious health issues that threaten your quality of life. In this chapter, I want to share several client success stories to illustrate why balanced blood sugar is so important.

Mary, forty-four, was a busy, more or less fit mom who came to see me because she wanted to shed ten pounds. As with many of my clients, we started simple: just begin each day with a Fab Four Smoothie, which is built with the Fab Four. Only ten days later, Mary looked and felt fantastic. She had dropped the ten pounds, was excited and confident about her body, and told me she wanted to train for a marathon. Woo-hoo!

Six months after completing the marathon, Mary called me for an appointment. She had joined a marathon training team and was training hard, but somehow she had gained more than fifteen pounds. She was also feeling terrible (drained, moody, apathetic) and was frustrated and confused by it all. I learned that her marathon training team had told her to add lots of "high-energy" carbohydrates, including sugary gels and energy bars, to her diet. Also, her training schedule was so demanding that she had stopped lifting weights and doing Pilates (which she had always done). I checked Mary's body fat percentage and it had gone up. I immediately suspected what had happened, so I sent her home with a glucometer to test and track her blood sugar. Sure enough, a week later we zeroed in on the issue: Mary was fighting chronically high blood sugar and potential insulin resistance.

Mary's training diet of "high-energy" carbohydrates had made her store the extra glucose as fat, causing her insulin levels to be through the roof. The macronutrients she was eating had caused both her weight gain and her negative moods. In addition, her muscle mass had decreased because she was no longer lifting weights or doing Pilates. It took a little time, but by returning Mary's diet to the Fab Four, consistently monitoring her blood sugar, and reintroducing muscle-building exercises to her regimen, we got her back. Back to a weight she was happy with, back to feeling energetic and happy, back to a place of balance.

Mary's case isn't unusual. When blood sugar is imbalanced, things can quickly go awry. It's not just extra pounds that get triggered, but potentially insulin resistance and metabolic syndrome, two conditions, like diabetes, that also stem from overproduction of insulin. As you might recall from chapter 2, insulin resistance is when your muscle cells don't respond to the "signal" from insulin and therefore don't accept glucose. As a result, more glucose stays in your bloodstream, raising your blood sugar. Over time, this can put you at risk for chronic high blood sugar (metabolic syndrome).

When people overeat starchy, processed, and simple carbohydrates at every meal without the balancing and slowing presence of fiber from vegetables, the pancreas begins to make too much insulin. Over time, when insulin levels are continually high, two things happen: (1) the pancreas gets worn out, and (2) cells become resistant to the "signal" from the insulin. (You can think of hormone tolerance like alcohol tolerance. Let's say you have a glass of wine every evening, Monday through Friday. By Friday, you might need three glasses of wine to give you the same chill vibes you had on Monday. Your body adjusts to the high level of sugar/alcohol and needs more for the "reward" to satisfy.) The result of all this? Week after week, month after month, year after year, such high levels of blood sugar and insulin float around your bloodstream, wreaking havoc and triggering insulin resistance and metabolic syndrome, which are always present when people are prediabetic or have been diagnosed with diabetes (type 1 or 2). When you double, triple, or quadruple spike your blood sugar at every meal, you're basically putting your body in a prediabetic state. One day it will break.

I've known Connie, thirty, since high school, when she was lean, strong, and athletic. As a college athlete, she started gaining weight and described herself as "swollen." After college, she got married and wanted to get pregnant. Her doctor looked at her hormone levels and diagnosed her with PCOS, which interferes with a woman's period and ovulation. The doctor then told her that she would not be able to conceive "naturally," and that she'd have to do in vitro fertilization (IVF) if she wanted to get pregnant. That's when she came to me.

Knowing that many cases of PCOS start with a high-sugar, high-carbohydrate diet, I asked Connie what she'd been eating. A sample day was oatmeal at breakfast, an apple as a snack, a sandwich for lunch, and then a dinner of chicken and rice. In Connie's case, the constant flow of insulin from her diet had created a type of insulin resistance that affected her ovulation, shutting down her body's hormonal cycle that would enable her to get pregnant. It had also caused her to gain weight and feel bloated.

I knew we needed to calm her body down so she could balance her sex hormones.

First we took the excess carbohydrates from her breakfast and lunch. She had a fruit-free Fab Four Smoothie to start the day; then for lunch she had a big salad loaded with veggies, protein (such as salmon or chicken), and fat (from olive oil and avocado). We moved her serving of carbohydrates (such as a sweet potato) to dinner to help increase her melatonin production so she could sleep. (Sleep is always good for your hormonal regulation!) After three months of my approach, she had lost twenty-two pounds (!) and was ready to make a baby "naturally," not through IVF. Within her first month of trying, she was pregnant! It brought us both to tears.

A high-sugar, high-starch, high-carbohydrate diet is also very taxing on your adrenal glands. This interferes with absorption of nutrients and causes weight gain. Your adrenal glands are located on top of your kidneys and are controlled by the pituitary gland in your brain. Their job is to help maintain stable blood sugar levels in your body during normal day-to-day activities.

When your blood sugar crashes, your adrenal glands release cortisol—the "stress hormone"—to help bring blood sugar back up. From the perspective of your adrenals, you're under stress and need more energy. Hence the cortisol—it increases your body's available blood sugar (indeed, it's the fight-or-flight mechanism hardwired into our brains and bodies that helps us stay alert to danger).

The problem is that overeating sugary and starchy foods can have us crashing down hard and relying on cortisol too often, as you'll be constantly signaling your adrenal glands to keep pumping out cortisol. Similar to the constant call for insulin, this constant call for cortisol eventually exhausts and fatigues the adrenal glands, making them function less. Over time, our bodies react to this constant stress by breaking down our immune systems, leaving us vulnerable to chronic fatigue, fibromyalgia, diabetes, and autoimmune diseases such as lupus. In addition, many people who have stressed adrenal functioning also have low thyroid function. Unfortunately, this is very common. The good news is that the Fab Four can help with both. My client Ashley, twenty-six, is an example.

I met Ashley on the set of a TV show when I was visiting another client. We began chatting, and she shared her juicing and vegetarian lifestyle with me. Although she didn't feel too bad at the time, I was concerned about her high-stress lifestyle; the high-sugar, high-soy diet she was on; and her lack of sleep. I cautioned her that the ups and downs, plus the phytoestrogen from soy, might be setting her up for hypothyroidism. To be frank, she sort of laughed in my face!

She called me three months later. She was in a bad place emotionally and physically. She was exhausted. She'd gained ten pounds, and her doctor had just prescribed her medicine for low thyroid function, caused (and compounded) by her diet of high carbohydrates, low fiber, and too much soy. I explained blood sugar balance to her and built her a mostly vegetarian plan full of high-fiber foods; healthy fats; and proteins such as eggs, beans, nuts, and seeds. She bounced back from her exhaustion, rediscovered her optimal weight, and sent me texts like these.

Zero hunger pretty much	12:13 PM
That's what I'm talking about!	12:13 PM
Randomly an egg white omelette with veggies and avo sounds good for lunch - eh?	12:20 PM
Yes!!! do it!!!	12:25 PM
Randomly?! body wants that protein	12:26 PM
Lolol	12:37 PM
Friday 1:48 PM	
They forgot my avo !!!	1:48 PM
I had 2 tbsp almonds with it !!	2:19 PM
You get it!! 🍴🍴	2:30 PM
Friday 6:29 PM	
0.000% hungry	6:29 PM
Food? Don't even need it	6:29 PM
Lol right?!	6:44 PM
Welcome to food freedom	6:44 PM

Another, sneakier way your blood sugar can become imbalanced is through *hidden* sugar in the foods you eat. Hidden sugar is *everywhere*—on every aisle at your typical grocery store, in processed foods, even in a lot of "clean, healthy" foods. Sometimes, though, the sugar is hidden in plain sight. Exhibit A: fruit.

Claire, forty-seven, was a serial fad dieter. She'd try going Mediterranean, Zone, vegan, pescatarian—you name it. She felt inflamed and wanted to get back into her skinny jeans. She was generally eating pretty clean—smoothies, kale salads, lots of fish, and so on. "So what's in your morning smoothie?" I asked her. "Frozen strawberries, almond milk and some protein powder," she responded. "How much fruit?" I probed. "Two cups or so," she said. That's too much fruit. I suggested that she use only $\frac{1}{4}$ cup of fruit for flavor, but more important, add 2 tablespoons of chia seeds (a fiber), plus 1 tablespoon of almond butter (a fat) and a handful of greens to keep her feeling full and balance her shake. She hesitated to add fat and calories, but she did it. A few days later, she texted me that she'd lost three pounds!

Claire isn't the only client who's been hesitant to add fat and calories. Many of my clients raise their eyebrows when I first tell them to add fat to their smoothie. But after just a few days, they see the effect fat and fiber have on their hunger levels, how it allows them to make better decisions at lunch and beyond.

More important, they trust their body to heal and go all in. That's when we achieve success—and sometimes a week is all it takes!

Claire's case is very common. We think fruit, which is natural, is chock-full of fiber, vitamins, and antioxidants. And this is true. But once digested, fruit breaks down into two sugars: glucose and fructose. You might recall from chapter 2 that fructose is metabolized 100 percent in the liver, turns into fat faster than other carbohydrates, and can potentially lead to a host of health issues. Generally, antioxidants combat free radicals (unstable molecules) in our bodies. But if there's too much fructose around, the body *super-oxidizes* free radicals, which results in liver inflammation and fatty liver disease, just like too much alcohol. Also, fructose can't be used effectively by your muscles and ends up shuffled over to your liver and synthesized as fat around your organs.

I'm sure you get these texts all the time but I have been making the Fab4 Smoothie and eating every 6 hours and I just lost 3 pounds! And finally broke a horrible habit of eating a zone bar every morning for years!! It's crazy because I have a history of an eating disorder and was very hesitant because of calories but it really works. And being post-menopausal it's hard to lose weight, but I did! For me at this point it is no longer just about how I look, it's more about how I feel and the smoothie helps me feel great!! Thank you!!

Blood sugar that is too high, too low, or wildly fluctuates between the two has negative effects throughout the body.

My friend's sixty-year-old father, Robert, came to me after getting a bad health report from his cardiologist. He didn't need to lose weight, but his numbers were bad (high cholesterol and inflammation) and signaled that he was at risk for a potential serious heart issue. He was a total athlete, worked out daily, and ate what he thought of as a "clean, all-American diet"—high-fiber cereal for breakfast; a sandwich for lunch; fruit, chocolate, or dried apricots for snacks; and a homemade dinner. He didn't drink much alcohol or eat saturated fat or red meat.

What was triggering his high cholesterol? The dried apricots that he munched on every day. His body was not breaking down the fructose. He had a continual flow of insulin and not enough healthy fat to combat the inflammatory omega-6 in his diet. We immediately pulled the dried fruit snacks, swapped his breakfast for a Fab Four Smoothie with coconut oil, and mandated a Fab Four lunch and dinner that included fish rich in omega-3 fatty acids. Within three months, Robert's blood tests showed no inflammation, and his cholesterol ratio returned to normal—and that was with an *increase* in saturated fat and cholesterol!

Too much fructose, like too much glucose, interferes with your hormonal functioning and your ability to feel satiated. If you don't feel full, your body will tell your brain you need more sugar. The current craze for agave-rich açaí bowls, date-sweetened smoothies, and juicing is the new "frozen yogurt," and they are making matters worse. These are all sources of extra sugar, specifically fructose. One popular diet among young women that includes a "green" smoothie actually suggests eating three different fruits for breakfast—apple, banana, and pear—but doesn't contain protein or fat (and it tops the charts at 25 grams of fructose). This is basically like starting your day with two glasses of rosé!

But I don't want you to ditch all your fruit. This is how to think about fruit: be aware of it, not afraid of it. Our bodies are made to eat fruit seasonally and occasionally. I'd keep it to one serving per day, in your smoothie, as dessert, or with a meal. As you will see in the coming chapters, my approach will allow you to enjoy fruit in ways that don't disrupt your blood sugar balance and trigger weight gain.

Liz, twenty-nine, came to me after having done the Whole30 program for a month with her boyfriend. She was frustrated that she had gained weight. "I stuck to the plan exactly—so why did I gain weight when my boyfriend lost almost fifteen pounds?" The problem was that she'd been starting her day with a package of cubed watermelon or pineapple from Trader Joe's. That high level of fructose in the morning spiked her blood sugar so aggressively that she was starving by lunch, in need of a snack at three P.M., and basically eating the rest of the day after that. She was up and down, hungrier than ever, and never feeling full. She was constantly eating—actually overeating—which caused her to gain weight (to the tune of six pounds).

Now, why did her boyfriend lose weight eating choices from the same program? Because, like most men, he wanted a savory breakfast of eggs and avocado instead of fruit. So his breakfast had little effect on insulin, and whatever glucose was in his bloodstream was sucked up by his lean muscle mass. Men on average are physically stronger and less affected by glucose, fructose, and other carbohydrates because of their hormone support (testosterone) and insulin-sensitive muscle mass.

IT'S UP TO YOU

I believe that the more you understand how food affects our bodies and brains, how our bodies break down food, and how food makes us function, the more likely you'll be to make the right choices for you. For me, this knowledge was power. It was what led me to form my company and develop the Fab Four. Even before that, it was what finally answered my never-ending list of questions. I needed to understand what was working and what wasn't, and why and why not. I hope this knowledge helps to liberate you from diets and scale jail, too.

It's my hope that no matter your situation, you will benefit from this book. At one end of the spectrum, there might be people who take food or dieting to an extreme. They may think "thin is in," starve themselves of proper nutrition to achieve a certain look, and prematurely age themselves. They may also be suffering from addiction, disorders, or other issues related to food. At the other side of the spectrum, there are people who ignore nutrition completely. They may be severely overweight, in a chronic state of bad health, and already dealing with food-related conditions such as high cholesterol, high blood pressure, diabetes, IBS, Crohn's disease, or breast or colon cancer. (And just to clarify—skinny people can have high cholesterol, too!) In reality, many of these ailments are *lifestyle* diseases that can develop from a lack of blood sugar balance.

Most of us live somewhere between the above extremes. Regardless of where you find yourself, the science tells us that if you eat clean, nutrient-dense forms of macronutrients, you will keep your blood sugar in balance, feel sated, and stop all sorts of health issues before they start. You'll balance your hormones, feel in control, and be empowered without having to exist in a fear-based state of vigilance. Most diets and regimens don't get to the root of the problem—lack of satiety, blood sugar imbalance, and hormonal disruption. My approach will set you free from the restrictive dietary noose and give you realistic, sustainable tools to live free and *be well!*

4
EMBRACING THE FAB FOUR FORMULA

THERE ARE COUNTLESS DIETS out there, and many of them in best-selling books. How do you know my approach is any different or better? And how do you know this approach to eating won't backfire and ultimately fail you, like diets may have in the past?

Well, first things first: This isn't a diet. It's not about deprivation, restriction, do-not-eat lists, or being forced to mentally fight cravings. It's a satisfying, realistic, and sustainable *lifestyle* that enables you to look and feel great, energized, and always in control. This is why so many different people have embraced my approach and had success with me—from actors, athletes, and executives to busy moms, work-aholics, and sugar junkies. My approach is different because it's livable, regardless of your background, and it's better because it uses science to get at the root of the problem—lack of satiety, blood sugar imbalance, and hormonal disruption.

As for backfiring and failing you? Nope, not gonna happen, for two main reasons.

First, by balancing your blood sugar, elongating your blood sugar curve, and keeping you satiated for up to six hours between meals, my approach sets your body up to do the work for you. Why? **Because you burn fat and lose weight in between meals (and during sleep) when your blood sugar is in balance and you don't have excess insulin in your bloodstream.** The research behind this is thorough, repeated, and clear: the key to reaching your healthy weight is through balancing your blood sugar and keeping your body in this metabolic state.

Second, my approach sets you up for long-term, sustainable success because it empowers you with the knowledge, understanding, and tools that diets don't. Diets are often short on all three and create more food drama in your life. My approach takes it away. You'll finally be free of worrying and obsessing about food and dieting because you'll understand how certain foods make you feel sated and good and how others make you crave and crash. You won't experience anxiety about your food choices.

And this means that cravings will go away, and instead you will discover a sense of incredible calm. You don't feel hungry. You aren't reaching for foods to soothe discomfort or emotional upset. And even if you indulge in some foods that spike your blood sugar for a day or two, you won't need to panic. You will autocorrect and reset your system so that you're right back in that softly swinging pendulum of balanced blood sugar. The result? Radiance, confidence, balance.

This is what I want for you—a *lifestyle* of balance that enables you to feel em-powered and not overwhelmed.

Once in balance, you will lose fat, increase lean muscle mass, and probably go down at least one jean size. Your hair will become thicker and shinier, your skin will clear up and take on a fresh glow, and your overall appearance will improve. On the inside, your body will adapt to this new inner balance by reducing pain and other inflammation, giving you more energy, and enabling you to sleep better. Over time, any illnesses that have crept up on you will be reversed, as your body adjusts to its natural homeostatic state.

Remember: You burn fat and lose weight **in between meals** (and during sleep), when your blood sugar is in balance and you don't have excess insulin in your bloodstream. That's why understanding *how* to achieve this balance is so important—the longer you can keep yourself in balance, the more weight you will lose and the more energy your body will have to do ongoing maintenance, so that you look and feel great.

Are you ready to shake and bake?

THE SIMPLICITY OF THE FAB FOUR FORMULA

One of my primary goals—next to helping you be well—is to help you eliminate all the self-doubt, uncertainty, and anxiety you might have surrounding eating and food choices. My formula does this by keeping it simple. It's straightforward, travels well, and easily helps you get right back on track if you feel out of balance. It's sustainable because it's easy to follow and actually livable. No rigid lists, complicated recipes, or crazy workouts.

My science-driven approach to eating relies on three simple actions:

1. Eat for satiety with the Fab Four and Fab Four Smoothie.
2. Elongate your blood sugar curve to burn fat.
3. Be "hormone aware" so you can autocorrect if necessary.

EAT FOR SATIETY

Whether it's your Fab Four Smoothie or other Fab Four breakfast or any other meal in your day, the Fab Four formula asks you to eat to satiety. What does that mean? Feeling satisfied and full without feeling stuffed or bloated. Basically, it's the calm you feel from a meal that does what it should: provide your body with the nourishment it needs. At a brain-body level, satiety is reached when your brain signals to your body that it has "enough" food. (Indeed, the word *satiety* comes from the Latin root *satis*, which means "enough.") Blood sugar and hormonal imbalances disrupt that signal and its effectiveness.

So what's "enough" food? Enough for *your* body. That's another reason a restrictive diet that prescribes certain amounts, portions, or number of calories typically backfires. We are all individuals with our own specific satiety markers. Most diets don't take this into account and end up leaving us wanting. We get up from one meal already thinking about the next. My approach will give you the right amount of "enough" for you.

And how do you regain sensitivity to your satiety? How do you retrain your body to let you know when it's full and has had enough? You get off that blood sugar roller coaster and balance your hunger hormones. Fewer big, crashing waves and more mellow rivers.

My approach doesn't just "ask you" to do all this. **The Fab Four formula is how you do it.** The specific combination of the Fab Four and the Fab Four Smoothie is designed to make you feel full and satisfied from the macronutrients your body wants and needs, and in a way that elongates your blood sugar curve. I repeat: eating the right proteins, fats, fibers, and greens is how you eat to satiety. When your body doesn't get these essential nutrients from the foods you choose, it provokes hunger and hormone imbalance, which cause you to eat more and more of the wrong things. On the other hand, eating the

the FAB FOUR

PROTEIN	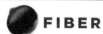 FAT	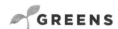 FIBER	GREENS
• signals to your brain that you're full. Protein increases production of GLP-1 (your "full" hormone), contributes to satiety due to its interaction with CCK (one of your "satiety" hormones), increases PYY (your "control" hormone), and releases dopamine (your "reward" hormone). (Also, a lack of protein increases NPY and "stimulates" your craving for more carbohydrates.) • contains B vitamins and minerals that help with overall food absorption. • is a source of amino acids, which builds blocks of cells and collagen for cell repair.	• increases satiety (through leptin and CCK). • reduces fasting insulin levels. • makes us feel calmer and more relaxed. • slows digestion. • curbs cravings. • maximizes loss of stored body fat (ketosis). • hydrates cells.	• provides food for good bacteria in the gut, which helps keep you regular. • helps the body produce butyrate, a short-chain fatty acid ("superfat" for the gut) that prevents cancer and has anti-inflammatory properties. • removes toxins from the body. • slows absorption of glucose.	• Produce antioxidants that repair cell damage from the environment. • Serve as anti-inflammatory, anticancer, and detoxification agents. • Provide naturally occurring resistant starch that feeds gut microbiota • Contain the sugar sulfoquino-vose that feeds gut microbiota. • Replace vitamins and minerals. • Offer medicinal properties for healing. • Provide phytonutrients and phytochemicals

Fab Four makes your body say: *"Got it, and thanks!"* Remember that hormone chart on pages 43–45? Each one of the Fab Four nutrients is specifically recommended at each meal for a reason! To help review, the chart above shows what these nutrient sources do for you.

BLUEBERRY MUFFIN

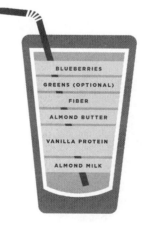

BLUEBERRIES
GREENS (OPTIONAL)
FIBER
ALMOND BUTTER
VANILLA PROTEIN
ALMOND MILK

FAB FOUR SMOOTHIE FORMULA

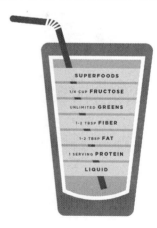

SUPERFOODS
1/4 CUP FRUCTOSE
UNLIMITED GREENS
1-2 TBSP FIBER
1-2 TBSP FAT
1 SERVING PROTEIN
LIQUID

The Blueberry Muffin Smoothie opposite provides an example of how these nutrients translate into a delicious Fab Four Smoothie breakfast.

63

Yum, right? (By the way, this recipe is just one of many knock-your-socks-off smoothies on the Fab Four plan. The delicious, wonderful-for-you Fab Four Smoothie recipes start on page 140. They're guaranteed to satisfy even the pickiest of eaters and always give you fun new options so you never get bored.)

As I mentioned earlier, I often recommend that new clients do nothing more than begin their day with a Fab Four Smoothie for breakfast for a week. When they experience the great flavor, satiety, and energy that comes with the Fab Four, they make a radical discovery: they're not starving by ten thirty A.M., they don't overeat a high-carb lunch, and they don't need sugary snacks to avoid a crash in the afternoon. I usually wake up to really cute (and surprised) texts that look like these:

iMessage
Today 4:30 PM

Hi Kelly! OMG I've lost 4 lbs!! Yay!! I was wondering. If I have coffee in the afternoon should I have it with coconut oil or almond milk?

Thank you so much for your help!! You are amazing

Don't you just love science?! Congrats on executing, that's a great amount of weight my dear! You can have it with either – if I were you I would have coconut oil because then I wouldn't be super hungry going into dinner and fat is free ♥ 👍

I am so proud of you!!! 😁 😁

But if you just ate almond milk would be my choice.

Okay awesome! Thank you so much!!!

Omg down another 1 1/2lbs 😱

3 1/5 total since last tues 💃💃💃💃💃💃💃

3 1/2

Hey girl heeeeeeeyyyyyy

These texts are why I love my job!!! It's science and not a fad, you shouldn't feel hungry or miserable. I am so proud of you and your commitment to wellness! You deserve every change on that scale!

If you have a breakfast meeting or can't have your Fab Four Smoothie for any reason, you can always use the Fab Four formula to build a breakfast. The smoothie is just a shortcut to the same great results. Either way, you'll feel full, balanced, and sated. Satiety gives you a great feeling of satisfaction throughout the day. When you start the day with a Fab Four Smoothie or a Fab Four meal, you do your body the favor of balancing your blood sugar with your very first meal. This will set you up to stop food cravings before they start and allow your body's natural metabolism to go to work (helping you burn fat and lose weight, if that's your goal). The calm and sense of fullness you'll feel is all the convincing you'll need in order to stick with the Fab Four and my approach.

ELONGATE YOUR BLOOD SUGAR CURVE

Beginning your day with balanced blood sugar sets you up to naturally hold on to and extend that sense of satiety for as long as possible. Another way I describe this is elongating your blood sugar curve. Your blood sugar will stay balanced within the "good range," you'll have fewer ups and downs, and the fluctuations will be less dramatic (no steep spikes or free-falling crashes). Eating to satiety "smoothens" out the curve and turns it into that longer, wavier line. The chart on the next page illustrates why that type of curve (as opposed to the crazy spike-crash version) helps you release fat, protect your lean muscle mass, eliminate cravings, and increase energy.

In addition, when you're eating meals with the Fab Four, you'll keep your blood sugar curve going *all on its own* so you don't have to stop to snack. So many of my clients lose their way on programs that require them to pick, buy, pack, and remember to carry extra snacks to get them from meal to meal. But when you eat to satiety, turn off hunger hormones, and elongate your blood sugar curve, you

BLOOD SUGAR CHART

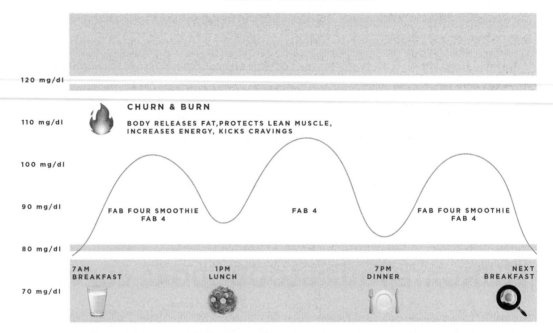

can skip this extra work and just go about your day. This is one of the many ways that my approach is different from other programs you may have tried.

I can hear you thinking, *How on earth can I go as long as six hours without feeling hungry?* Many of my new clients have that same question, followed by this one: *Don't I need to stoke my metabolism by eating every three hours?* No. The research shows that eating so frequently is actually unhealthy and detrimental to weight loss goals. The latest endocrine science tells us that eating every three or four hours actually sets us up for not only *exhaustion* and *premature aging*, but also *less fat burning*. Why? When you eat, you begin the process of digestion, which requires your body to expend a lot of time and energy to break down food into molecules that can be absorbed and utilized. Complete digestion usually takes six hours or more. When you eat snacks between meals, you tax your body. You are asking it to restart a process it has not yet completed from the last time you ate. Not only does this take energy away from other repairs your body is making (hello, tired eyes), but it also *adds pounds*. When your body cannot absorb and utilize food, it stores it as fat. In addition, restarting the process of digestion cuts short your body's ability to burn fat in between meals, when blood sugar is in balance. That's the power of being in blood sugar balance: you can actually burn fat.

Eating for satiety and elongating blood sugar balance enables you to metabolize fat in between meals, not just when you sleep. Your Fab Four Smoothie lets you start your day in a balanced blood sugar state and burn fat in between breakfast and lunch. Then, when you follow this breakfast with two other nutrient-rich meals, you elongate your blood sugar curve for more of the same between lunch and dinner. You don't get cravings, you stay calm and centered, and you can trigger your body to lose weight (if that's what you want).

Essentially, you are retraining your body how to feel full and satisfied and find its optimal weight all on its own, without interference from a diet that relies on calorie counting and restriction.

BE HORMONE AWARE

By eating to satiety and establishing a smoother, less erratic blood sugar curve throughout the day, you're also keeping your hunger hormones regulated and on an even keel. From this place, you learn to consciously connect with how your body is feeling and what it might need to stay in blood sugar balance. This is what I call making yourself "hormone aware." The more balanced you are, the more clearly you will know when you need to eat and when you don't.

Remember the interplay between insulin (released when you eat carbohydrates), ghrelin (your "hunger" hormone), and leptin (your "I'm full" hormone)?

After a big meal, you shouldn't be hungry. But when your bloodstream is full of insulin, you can *feel* hungry an hour after a meal (if not sooner) and start looking for a snack or wanting to graze. That isn't real hunger; it's hormonal hunger.

When you make yourself "hormone aware," you will be able to **read what your body is telling you** about what is happening with your blood sugar balance. When you're balanced, hunger isn't immediate. You'll feel your metabolism kick in, but it's slower and comes on gradually, a product of your satiety and elongated blood sugar curve. By contrast, when you're not balanced, you'll experience sudden and strong cravings, maybe even with a headache and a steep drop in energy on the side. You'll feel anxious and be tempted (because of your hormones) to grab for sugary, processed foods to fix it. Being hormone aware means you understand and know how to respond to your body's unique signs for high and low blood sugar.

Healthy weight loss happens **between meals** when we have balanced blood sugar and no excess insulin. It happens when our leptin, ghrelin, and other hormones are communicating with one another. Understanding blood sugar and being aware of your hormones is a great way to facilitate long-term healthy fat loss. In addition, it can help keep your metabolism working at its maximum efficiency and prolong satiety. When you eat for satiety, giving your body the right combination of protein, fat, fiber, and greens, your body expends less energy for digestion and increases your metabolism. It works like a high-tech machine without any glitches.

DITCH PERFECTION

For Lisa, twenty-seven, a bachelorette weekend took its toll. By Sunday she was craving pizza, felt lethargic and puffy, and was up a few pounds. My suggestion was to have a smoothie dinner for a few nights at the beginning of the week, then make sure her lunches were Fab Four meals. This helped bring down her inflammation, high blood glucose, and cravings by Thursday, no harm done. (See page 231 for more easy, simple autocorrect strategies!)

None of us is perfect. Perfection isn't even real. It's an unreasonable, unattainable, and self-destructive standard to hold yourself to. Being **hormone aware** lets you ditch the inevitable disappointment from trying to be perfect and quickly "autocorrect" if you've eaten something that doesn't agree with you (or your goals!) or takes you out of balance. You'll trust your body's signals and simply add food for additional satiety and a longer blood sugar curve.

> Just sent 💰 via PayPal. Thank you again for organizing everything. Btw, I have lost 4lbs since Monday. Only did smoothie for breakfast and dinner on Monday but have had them everyday for breakfast. You're a miracle worker and I love you to pieces. I always forget how full they make me and I am not FAMISHED by lunchtime. And it sets the tone for the whole day. Not telling you anything you don't already know! Thanks boo 😘😘
>
> Sure do!!
>
> See you tonight!!
>
> What did I tell you!! Congrats!! You put in the hard work and it paid off. 🖤
>
> Delivered

PART TWO

THE
FAB FOUR
SOLUTION

5
KNOWING YOURSELF

BEING IN CONTROL OF your body isn't just about knowing what to eat and when and why. It's also about *knowing yourself*. This is an extension of my holistic philosophy, one that takes into account the whole you—your mental, emotional, psychological, and social makeup. So in order to leverage the full power of my approach, let me ask you a few questions: What is going on in your life? What internal or external pressures are you feeling? What do you want? Why do you want it? What has "derailed" you in the past? What's holding you back mentally?

A lot of my clients get the science and adopt the Fab Four pretty quickly. It's everything else connected to food that takes time and effort to break through.

Indeed, a huge part of my job goes beyond nutrition advice and counseling. I'm a friend, a coach, a confidante, and a therapist. Food is emotional, and no matter how well you're doing you're bound to encounter one challenge or another. You're human. A living, breathing, thinking, and *feeling* being. Sometimes our thoughts and feelings can get the best of us. Life happens. Things may rise to the surface, you might come face-to-face with emotions you used to eat your way through, past "failures" might rear their heads. And changing old habits, negative attitudes, or self-defeating thought processes takes time.

You'll feel much more energetic, vibrant, and in sync with yourself when you adopt the Fab Four lifestyle, but there will be hurdles to clear. What follows is a Fab Four toolkit of sorts to help you as you make this shift. I want you to better understand yourself so that you recognize when you're holding yourself back and know what to do. Here are the simple tools that will help you build confidence, trust, and peace from within.

TOOL #1: WHAT'S YOUR "WHY"?

Why did you pick up this book? What are you looking for? Why is that motivating to you?

I love inspirational quotes, stories, and people. My personal guilty pleasure guru is Tony Robbins. His voice resonates with me, and I find that his mind-set and philosophy cut through the noise and help me get in touch with what really matters. My number one takeaway from Mr. Robbins? **That we are in control of our lives.** Truly. We can steer its course and shape its outcomes, even when something unexpected happens. But for that kind of navigation, we need to be clear at the outset **why we're doing what we're doing.**

So let's start with your why.

Why are you here? What is it that you want to do differently? This isn't just some hippie-dippie exercise. Purpose drives us. By asking (and answering) yourself, you'll begin the process of forging a powerful "emotional logic" between your why and the foods you eat. You're consciously connecting your **deeper purpose** to your **daily decisions.** It's the start of a bond, a pact, with yourself. It will increase your likelihood of success, give you inner strength, and propel you forward through any bumps or obstacles.

Your why may not be immediately clear to you and might take you some digging inside of yourself. Take my client Kerry, forty-seven, for example. Kerry is a pistol. She works full time (as does her husband), has three teen and tween daughters, and is a social butterfly. Her life is frenetic, fun, and fabulous. She travels for work, drives her girls around on the weekends, and, in between, tries to have some hubby time. She also loves to get together with her girlfriends. Unfortunately, she never has a moment to chill. I get tired just listening to how busy she is!

Over the past few years, as Kerry hit her mid-forties, she gained about twenty-five pounds. At first she told herself the extra weight didn't bother her, but it did. She couldn't wear a lot of her favorite clothes and felt embarrassed in her bathing suit. She had also slowly withdrawn from her husband because she felt frumpy and unattractive.

Kerry's why? "At first, my why seemed to be that I just wanted to lose weight. I thought losing twenty pounds would make all my problems disappear. But as I got started and dropped the first five pounds, I realized that it was more complicated than that. I had lost touch with me, at my core. My life had become so busy and I no longer knew how to take care of myself. I know I have to slow down, that I'm trying to do too much. But I think I run at hyperspeed just so I can avoid myself."

Kerry is so not alone. Her deeper why—to reconnect with herself—is something I think we all can relate to. And understanding it became a powerful motivator for her. After just two weeks beginning her day with a Fab Four

Smoothie, Kerry lost twelve pounds. "I'm not thirty-two anymore, but I feel so much better than I did last month, and that's a start," she explained. "What losing that first five and then ten pounds did was connect *me* to *me*—that's what I was missing and that's what I have refound." At one time, making a smoothie might've been just another thing on Kerry's endless to-do list. But her why helped turn it into a ritual with deeper meaning, thus setting her up for success.

Here are some other whys that my clients have shared with me. Maybe they will inspire you. (And if your why is only physical at this point, that's totally fine. Your why is what it is. The point is to be open and honest with yourself!)

"Better overall health, better blood tests, and longevity."

"Less bloating (and gas) and more regularity."

"Solve my gut or food intolerance issue, so I can *enjoy* food again."

"Clear up my skin and get that supple, healthy, glowing look."

"Stop obsessing and stressing over food. I want to trust myself!"

"Live free of scale anxiety and constantly worrying about how much I weigh."

"Accept myself and my body, and rock it!"

"Get stronger and look toned."

"More energy, please! Just more energy so I can thrive each and every day."

"Be able to run around the block or take a yoga class without being embarrassed about my jiggly bits, so I can work out consistently."

"Lose weight, specifically these love handles."

"Fit into a smaller size jean."

"Bikini body all year."

"Play longer with my nieces and nephews."

"Love myself and stop the negative self-talk."

Many of these whys may resonate with you. You also might discover that your why is something deeper, more emotional or spiritual. Like Kerry, you might just find a deep connection with yourself and light the path of taking care of yourself again.

TOOL #2: SET REALISTIC GOALS

Knowing your why unlocks the door, but then what? How do you pursue it?

When making health and lifestyle changes, the "how" is often its own source of anxiety. This is because your past hows—aka *diets*—are still in your system. They come with mental baggage, old scars, and self-inflicted wounds. Indeed, even as you think about shifting away from counting calories and obsessing about food to living a Fab Four lifestyle that enables you to enjoy food and empowers you to be self-reliant, it's very easy to get frightened. It's also easy to second-guess yourself; get distracted by self-doubt; think about every time you've tried a diet and "failed;" heap extra pressure on yourself; grow impatient because you want it all *right now*; and set goals that are unrealistic. The judgment, the shame, the doubt—it all stems from the **ghosts of diets past** and the mind-set that we can't control our health, well-being, and food. It's time to forgive yourself for living under the weight of self-judgment. It's time to press delete, swipe left, and not let what's in the rearview mirror control you anymore.

So how do you do this? What's the first step?

By setting **realistic goals** for yourself right out of the gate. Instead of imagining goals of losing thirty pounds in one month or competing in your first triathlon in three months, keep your goals simple and attainable. Goals should still be goals—things you want to strive and push yourself to achieve. But setting realistic goals will help you build self-confidence, trust in yourself and the process, and manage your own expectations. My approach is realistic because that's what it asks of you. This concept is built into my approach, which is why it has helped so many different people build their own healthy, sustainable *lifestyle*.

I often rely upon the scientifically supported and very popular (because it works!) "SMART" goals framework (first developed in 1981 by managing consultant George T. Doran) to help my clients envision goals that they can be most successful at. You want to decide on a **Specific** goal that you can **Measure** (or track), that is **Achievable** given your present circumstances, that is meaningful and **Relevant** to you, and that is realistic based upon your **Time frame**.

Experts on motivation and achievement define SMART goals as:

- Be **specific**. If getting in shape and losing weight is your general goal, decide specifically what that means by using a body-loving measure that reflects *your* body, such as dropping one jean size, decreasing your body fat percentage by X percent, increasing your muscle mass by Y percent, or being able to rock that one dress, suit, or

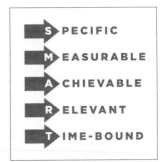

bathing suit in your closet. Pounds are everyone's default, but try to make it specific in another way.

- Next, ask yourself how to make that goal **measurable**. You need a system that tracks your progress. If your goal is losing a jean size, then measuring your waist is a good way to measure your progress. If your goal is to reduce sugar in your diet because you want to get rid of cravings, then writing down all the foods you eat each week will help you research how much sugar is in each, then compare yourself week to week. (Tool #5 suggests that you keep a Fab Four Notebook that keeps you tracking not only your goals, but also how you are feeling. It can be in the notes on your smartphone, through a blog that you write for yourself, or in an old-fashioned black-and-white marble notebook!)

- Make sure that your goal is **achievable** given your present circumstances and where you're at in your life. For instance, if my client Kerry's goal had been to lose twenty-five pounds in one month, she would likely been setting herself up for failure and disappointment. Instead, her specific goal was to lose two pounds this week—much more realistic given her time frame. (And she exceeded her goal! She lost the first twelve pounds in two and half weeks!)

- Is your goal meaningful and **relevant** to your life? This step connects back to your why. My tip is to think about *long-term* relevancy. Why do you want to lose weight? Why do you want to cut out processed foods? Why do you want to get in shape? If you're temporarily motivated to get into your bikini for a vacation, what happens when you're back from the trip? However, if you want to get in shape so that you feel more confident in your own skin, no matter the setting, then you're making a deeper kind of connection that will have staying power.

- Finally, you want to establish a **time frame** that works for you. This is what making your goal time-bound means. Setting a timeline for your goal helps you plot out how to get there. Instead of having your goal be attached to some vague and distant future, your time frame will help you stay focused and motivated on reaching your goal.

The SMART framework is one of many tools out there to help ensure your goals are realistic. If another methodology, or none at all, works better for you, then use it. The point is to help ease your transition to balance by converting lofty, ambitious desires into more manageable, concrete goals.

WHAT ARE YOUR GOALS?

Now, before you write down fifty SMART goals and try to change your whole entire life again, let's prioritize! Write down ten realistic goals you want to achieve, then put them in order of importance to you.

1. Do you have wellness goals?
   - More energy?
   - Better sleep?
   - Decreased dependency on medicines?
2. Do you have weight-loss goals?
   - What amount of weight can you realistically expect to lose in one week? Two weeks? Start small and build toward an ultimate goal.
   - What is your ideal weight?
3. Do you have lifestyle goals?
   - To exercise more frequently?
   - To explore exercise options (i.e., try something new!)?
   - Are you interested in adding some mindfulness relaxation as a stress reliever?

By identifying your goals in concrete ways, following up in ways that are measurable and attainable, you will soon make all of the microsteps into life-long habits. That's how you make being well sustainable lifestyle!

Pushing yourself to achieve goals is a great way to build confidence in your abilities and bolster your self-esteem. Any time you show up for yourself, it's a touchdown and will motivate you for the next time—whether that's showing up to a spin class, starting your day with a Fab Four Smoothie, or building your own Fab Four menu. Each time you move toward your goal is a win. You're showing yourself that you are in control of your life . . . life is not in control of you! Just remember to be realistic!

TOOL #3: SHIFT YOUR MIND-SET

Tuning into yourself and your why, and writing down realistic goals, are both steps toward building a Fab Four lifestyle, but you also have to *believe* that it's possible to make these changes.

One of the main challenges of my job is helping my clients shift their mind-set regarding food. They're often stuck in a negative, self-defeating headspace in which they don't believe in themselves. It's usually the by-product of a long and tortured relationship with food, rife with all sorts of subconscious land mines from past diets. I try to eliminate that self-doubt and replace it with self-belief by coaching my clients to take one positive action in the direction of their goal, one meal or situation at a time.

The typical diet mentality is that you're only ever "on" or "off" plan. This is why one little "mistake" can have such devastating consequences. *I screwed up at lunch. Now the whole day is ruined.* You hold yourself to an impossible standard (perfection), and when you inevitably don't meet it, all is lost for the day, weekend, or week ahead (failure). Next thing you know, you're backsliding, bingeing, and beating yourself up. For many of us, this cycle of self-defeat is an ingrained pattern.

I coach my clients to acknowledge when they feel one of these cycles coming on and to counteract it by taking one positive action in the direction of their goal. Action will erase the anxiety and immediately reinforce that you're in control. It doesn't have to be something big. It can be sending a text to your partner about dinner plans, or supporting your body with a lap around the office or a glass of water, or maybe checking your blood sugar to educate yourself about how your body is reacting. Sometimes the little picture *is* the big picture. One decision—your next—is all that matters. It's looking out at life through the windshield, not the rearview mirror, and ditching the things that drag you down and hold you back—judgment, shame, self-doubt. *"That piece of cake happened. And it was delicious. But I know I'll feel a bit off in the morning. I better plan on a smoothie to balance me out."*

Stanford University psychologist and researcher Carol Dweck has written extensively about turning limiting beliefs around so that you can reframe challenges as opportunities and setbacks as simply information, not judgments about what you can or cannot do, or your value as a person. Dweck has shown that we either believe our intelligence is preset (and thus our success is based on innate ability) or believe intelligence can be developed or grown over time (and thus our success is based on hard work, learning, and perseverance). Dweck refers to these two attitudes as fixed and growth-oriented. A person with a fixed mind-set believes that a setback or mistake means they're not good or smart enough. A person with a growth-oriented mind-set takes those things as feedback, to try harder or do something different.

How does this relate to you? If you've tried a hundred diets, lost weight, and then gained it back, you might secretly believe it's your fault—that you simply can't lose weight and sustain that weight loss. That would be an example of a fixed mind-set. On the other hand, you might believe that you just haven't discovered the approach that works for you, but that you will eventually persevere. That's the growth-oriented mind-set. You can guess what camp I fall into! Have I been frustrated and self-blaming in the past? Yes, but I also always believed that I'd discover a way to **be well** that was right for me. The Fab Four is that plan.

I've adapted Dweck's suggestions for shifting your mind-set from fixed to growth-oriented with these steps:

1. **IDENTIFY AND ACKNOWLEDGE SELF-DEFEATING THOUGHTS.**
   They all come from a place that change is impossible; that you cannot learn or grow; that you are predetermined to be where you are now. And all that will be true unless you shift your mind-set.
2. **REMEMBER THAT YOU HAVE THE POWER** to disregard those thoughts and instead think of yourself as someone who is absolutely able to grow and make changes. All it takes is a willingness to try, some effort, and a belief that it's possible.
3. **REINFORCE YOUR GROWTH-ORIENTED CHOICE.** For example, write in your Fab Four Notebook or remind yourself of all the other Fab Four

peeps who are making the change, too. If they can do it, so can you! And remember, this is not about perfection. With a growth mind-set, we take any setbacks at face value and learn from them.

4. **MAKE IT REAL.** Acknowledge the challenges you face, your discomfort and disappointment, but without personalizing it or blaming yourself. Think of each challenge—big or small—as an opportunity to grow and learn more about yourself. If you feel out of balance, ask yourself, What's the lesson here? Why was this day or weekend or week so hard for me? And finally, take responsibility, not by judging yourself as a failure, but by *taking action* in the direction of your goal.

It's possible to lose weight and not put it back on. It's possible to stabilize your blood sugar, eat meals that make you feel full and satisfied, and lose weight at the same time. It's possible not only because the research says so but also because I have seen numerous people make these small changes to the way they eat and discover an amazing new life for themselves.

TOOL #4:
KNOW HOW *YOUR* BODY REACTS

The concept of **bio-individuality** is important to keep in mind as you embark on your journey to find balance. The fundamentals of my approach—eating to satiety with the Fab Four, elongating your blood sugar curve, and balancing your hunger hormones—are rooted in nutritional science and how the human body works. Bio-individuality takes into account each person's inherent differences and unique needs for nutrition and how we each might respond differently to certain foods.

Although we all need the basic building blocks of nutrition (nutrient-dense macronutrients), some of us can process more carbohydrates because we have more lean muscle mass, and some of us gain two pounds just looking at a bowl of pasta. These different kinds of variability are due to a combination of our current health (including weight, height, and muscle mass), our genes, our personal history (such as our behaviors), and the environment in which we live. Understanding how your body responds to certain foods, exercise, and lack of sleep is important to monitor and track, so you can adjust your lifestyle as need be.

For example, not only am I celiac (allergic to the protein in wheat), but I also recently discovered that I am intolerant of dairy—I began to notice stomach upset after eating certain kinds of dairy. I confirmed my suspicions when I did a Cyrex IgE food allergy test done with Los Angeles–based functional medicine physician Dr. Apostolos Lekkos. This knowledge of how *my* body reacts has informed my food decisions. I don't use whey protein in my Fab Four Smoothie (whey is a dairy product), opting instead for a great-tasting pea plant protein powder.

Food allergies, intolerances, and leaky gut are real. We can see the reactions through blood tests, elimination testing, and allergy testing. (I get food allergy tests every two to three years to check out what is going on inside my body.) Some of you may need to remove gluten, dairy, soy, or even FODMAPS (fermentable oligosaccharides, disaccharides, monosaccharides and polyols). FODMAPS, a group of short-chain carbohydrates and sugar alcohols naturally contained in foods or food additives, such as fructose, fructans, galacto-oligosaccharides (GOS), lactose, and polyols (e.g., sorbitol and mannitol), are poorly digested and can lead to IBS. My approach is about keeping your gut well and thriving by consuming probiotics and prebiotic fiber and removing chemicals, allergens, and GMOs.

Jen, thirty-two, was suffering from acne, bloating, and strong acid reflux. Two of the main triggers for these reactions are gluten (the proteins found in wheat—gliadins and glutenins) and dairy (typically because of lactose, but also due to casein and whey). Jen was adamant that she did not have an issue with either, but in fact she had a pretty strong addiction to them. She seemed almost mad that I wanted to try taking them away, but after a twenty-one-day elimination period, we brought back gluten and dairy individually and she became sick again, with painful and debilitating cramps.

Sometimes it's not so cut-and-dried. You might not experience a dramatic reaction to a food that is causing an issue in your body. To determine with certainty, you have to cut it out and see how you feel. Jen isn't missing any nutrition leading a gluten- and dairy-free life now, but she is missing about twenty pounds she used to carry!

Aria, twenty-nine, is a manager at a fitness club and is in awesome shape. She eats a mainly vegetarian diet with some fish every now and then. Sounds clean, right? Yet she suffered from a stubborn case of severe acne. When we looked at everything she was eating during her typical day and week, we found one culprit: soy. Her morning coffee order was a soy latte. Her lunch was often a macrobiotic bowl based around tofu, which is made from soybeans. I encouraged her to pull the soy, and within about six weeks, her acne significantly improved. What hidden culprit are you relying on each day?

You might already know if you are sensitive to gluten, dairy, or soy, but if not, use these questionnaires to see if you might be reactive.

Gluten Questionnaire
Do you suffer from any of the following:

- frequent bloating or gas?
- IBS or acid reflux?
- daily or regular diarrhea, or chronic constipation?
- migraines or headaches?
- joint pains or aches?

- forgetfulness or brain fog?
- depression or anxiety?
- ADD or ADHD now or as a child?
- low thyroid?
- eczema or acne?

Dairy (Lactose, Whey, or Casein) Questionnaire
Do you suffer from any of the following:

- nausea, diarrhea, bloating, or flatulence?
- IBS?
- acne, itchy skin, or eczema?
- mood swings, or have you been diagnosed with depression?
- respiratory problems like coughing, asthma, or sinusitis?

Soy Questionnaire
Do you suffer from any of the following:

- hormonal acne?
- low thyroid?
- fatigue?
- slow BM motility?

If you suffer from two or more conditions in any one category of food, consider cutting that category from your diet for four to six weeks to see if you have a food allergy or intolerance. If so, I recommend getting tested immediately; depending on the open-mindedness of your health care adviser, he or she might provide such tests. Insurance coverage varies by company. You can always seek out a functional medicine provider, who practices a more holistic approach and often provides these tests.

TOOL #5: GET TESTED

One other way to know your own chemistry and how you might need to tweak the Fab Four and Fab Four Smoothie is to monitor your blood sugar. If you feel like you tend to vacillate and it's hard for you to reach that "gentle roll" on the blood sugar curve, you might benefit from getting a metabolic panel, which will include glucose, A1C, and other factors that will help you understand your overall blood sugar level.

But keep in mind that the results can be deceiving because they don't show you what your blood sugar curve actually looks like on a day-to-day (or hour-to-hour) basis. As the diagram shows below, two drastically different curves can have a very similar "average."

One curve stays within range, while the other is a wild roller coaster of

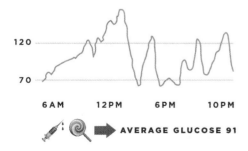

MAY 2016
REGULAR HEALTHY LIFESTYLE

120
70

6AM   12PM   6PM   10PM

AVERAGE GLUCOSE 91

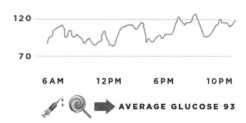

JUNE 2016
FAB FOUR LIFESTYLE

120
70

6AM   12PM   6PM   10PM

AVERAGE GLUCOSE 93

spikes and crashes. It's important to keep in mind that getting the A1C is a good step, but it can be erroneous as an indicator. For example, if you look at the two diagrams above, the person with the 93 has ostensibly higher blood sugar, but he also has a much more balanced curve over time. The person on the right with the so-called lower blood sugar shows dramatic spikes throughout the day. So one test of your blood sugar is often not enough to get a reliable, complete understanding of whether your blood sugar is indeed high or low, or spiky or more balanced, which is why going to the doctor once for a blood sugar screening may not be enough. If you buy a home test, you can test your blood sugar more often and develop a more complete picture of your levels. (See below for more on how to interpret your own body signals and make adjustments to your diet.)

INTERPRETING YOURSELF

How do you feel? This may seem like a simple question, but it's also a very important one. In order to maximize the impact of eating as outlined in this book, you need to know when and how to tweak your Fab Four meals or Fab Four Smoothie, and this requires you to pay attention to your own signals—both physical and emotional. Take a look at these three different people and how they made slight changes to the Fab Four formula because of their individual needs, including those who relied upon the use of glucometer to better track their blood sugar throughout the day.

Davina, a twenty-seven-year-old artist, wanted to lose fifteen to twenty pounds. At five foot ten, Davina is big-boned and athletic. Her goal was not to become rail thin, but she had gained about twenty pounds since she'd stopped playing volleyball after college, and now her doctor was telling her she was insulin resistant and showing signs of metabolic syndrome. After two weeks of eating on my plan, she'd lost eight pounds. "But," she confessed to me, "I feel irritable and anxious."

Those words—*irritable* and *anxious*—are typical signs that someone's blood sugar is too low. First, I made sure that Davina was using the full smoothie recipe of 2 tablespoons of fiber and 2 tablespoons of fat (such as MCT oil and/or avocado). She was, but not every day. So I suggested that Davina add 10 more grams of protein powder to her morning smoothie and also add in a fat-protein snack (almond butter packet or coconut almond butter packet) in the late afternoon before dinner. When Davina made these two adjustments, she continued to lose weight (3 or 4 pounds a week), and she felt much more settled and calm.

But I really wanted Davina to feel connected to her body and reach a strong peace of mind, so I suggested that she use a glucometer for a couple of weeks to get used to the way her body began to shift its metabolism. That way, she could time her snacks and meals more appropriately. After a few weeks, she didn't need to test herself anymore. She had learned to understand her body.

Leslie, forty-two, is an executive at a Fortune 500 company in a high-stress, very demanding job. She came to me to lose weight and because she was fatigued and in a constant state of high anxiety and just didn't feel like herself. She rises early, gets to work by seven thirty A.M., and often works late, past seven P.M., starting and ending her day in traffic—L.A. life! After consulting with me, she had her Fab Four Smoothie for breakfast, and then at about noon, she went to the company cafeteria for lunch and had a salad with chicken and veggies or an omelet. By the time she headed home, it was almost seven P.M. and she was starving, so she'd stop at Whole Foods and pick up a great Fab Four meal— salmon sashimi and a couple of good side dishes. After several months, Leslie had lost twenty-four pounds.

Her mistake? She'd be so hungry that she'd eat her dinner on the way from the grocery store. By the time she got home, she'd "finished" dinner. She ate so quickly that her brain and body had not even registered the food—either physically (her brain couldn't keep up with its satiety signals) or emotionally (so she found herself snacking through the night). So as with Davina, I suggested a mandatory bridge snack—a protein and fat combo (such as half an avocado, a packet of mixed nuts, or a Roadie, a small Fab Four Smoothie you can take on the go) that would settle her down. As soon as Leslie started to incorporate a bridge snack around five P.M., she was calm enough to wait to get home to eat, and she didn't find herself snacking on Glutino pretzels at odd hours of the night! Her body adapted quickly and easily to this new routine, so she didn't feel the need to use a glucometer to test or track her blood sugar; she knew she was in good balance when she wasn't "caving and craving."

Thirty-nine-year-old entrepreneur Tyler had high blood pressure, adrenal fatigue, and signs of metabolic syndrome. He came to me after his doctor said he could reverse his pre-diabetes and high blood pressure through good nutrition and regular exercise. Like many of us, Tyler would start his day with a latte or nothing at all and often work through lunch. It would suddenly be three P.M. and he'd have a migraine and feel queasy and dizzy. I explained that he was pushing his body too far. He needed to eat lunch in order to keep himself in balanced blood sugar without taxing his adrenals. So we did two things: we made sure his assistant ordered a clean lunch for him, which he had to sit down and eat before one P.M.; and he began to use his glucometer after he'd eaten and then later in the evening before dinner. He discovered in a very specific way how his blood sugar would drop and spike if he did not stick to his plan. And although I couldn't convince him to give up his latte, I got him to add in a breakfast Fab Four Smoothie first thing in the morning to support his adrenals. He also started testing his blood sugar first thing in the morning (fasting) and testing again one to two hours after each meal (post-prandial). Our plan helped Tyler gain concrete feedback about where he was on his curve and how specific foods affected him.

In general, men need 6 to 8 ounces of protein per meal, whereas women need 4 to 6 ounces of protein. However, depending on your shape, amount of muscle mass, and how frequently you exercise, you might need more protein and more fat with your meals. If you begin to feel shaky or tired in the afternoon, add a side of avocado to your lunch. If that doesn't work, give yourself a **bridge snack** of protein plus fat, such as a hard-boiled egg or a small amount of grass-finished beef jerky, or tuna or salmon salad. And by all means, if you think your blood sugar is not evening out and you continue to feel sharp drops and spikes in blood sugar over the course of the day, then consult your physician and request the A1C test, knowing that you might need to repeat the test to really understand your average range. You might also benefit from using a glucometer until you've figured out how best to stay in balance throughout the day.

TOOL #6: TRACK YOURSELF

Throughout this process, it's crucial to check in with yourself and stay connected with how you feel physically, emotionally, and mentally. As I mentioned earlier, I recommend that you keep a Fab Four Notebook in your phone, on your computer, or in a journal. You'll be tracking not only your goals but how you are feeling, hour by hour and day by day. As you stay aware of how you feel, you'll begin to tie it to the foods you are eating. Remember, the goal is to be **hormone aware**. This will help you stay attuned not only to reactions you might be having but also to your dips in mood, including any moments when you might slip back into a fixed mind-set.

Believe me, I know how hard it is to stay motivated. After a long holiday weekend of letting a few things slide, you can feel even less motivated to get back on track. You probably have a high fasting blood sugar number that you need to whip back into shape, plus a little residual inflammation, and those sugary choices have probably been messing with your sleep. For most of my clients, tracking works as a great way to stay self-connected, learn how to autocorrect, and bounce back from any slip-ups.

Here's what to include in your notebook:

- Your SMART goals, including progress, successes, setbacks, and challenges
- Your thoughts, feelings, and moods, not only about food but about your life in general
- Your meals and snacks
- Your exercise, sleep, and other activities

IF YOU'RE A BIT TYPE A . . .

An important note: If you're extremely type A and have a tendency to obsess, regret, and self-punish over food decisions, tracking can potentially exacerbate those issues. If you fall into this camp, I recommend that you don't track yourself. Instead, trust yourself. Take a look at the case studies starting on page 99 and learn how to check in with yourself and trust your body's signals. Do you need more protein or fat? Are you feeling a bit stopped up and sluggish? Do you need a bit more fiber? These cues can be useful to you even if you don't write everything down in a Fab Four Notebook.

CLAIM YOUR HAPPY PLACE

I consider myself a happy person. One of my biggest joys in life is to make other people happy. Just ask my husband. I like to smile, laugh out loud, and make every situation as fun as possible. This sunny disposition has helped me a lot in life. But we all have our good days and our bad, our ups and our downs. That's life. The more we accept these ebbs and flows instead of fighting them and judging ourselves, the more we can move through our emotions productively. I'm a big fan of having a cry and moving on, not reliving or dwelling on things, and not putting myself through unnecessary emotional torture.

When we embrace that we are always changing—our identity, our bodies, our brains, our relationships, our work—then we can become more loving toward ourselves. Instead of judging how we feel or don't feel, we can simply be aware of our feelings, accept them, and choose to stay in that happy place.

Being truly well comes from committing to this happy place. Replace the dopamine spike you get from sugar with music, exercise, touch, laughing, or setting a realistic goal. (Yep, time to set that SMART goal!) When your body feels better through non-food-related rewards, it's easier to be calm and mindful. We will always encounter challenges, distractions, pain, and even loss. But remember, breakthroughs often come through these times of adversity. And when these curve balls come our way, we can use our relationship with our own happy place to find solace and strength from within, instead of from unhealthy food or other behaviors that do us harm.

6

YOUR FAB FOUR MEALS AND RECIPES

SO WHAT WILL YOU be eating? Let's begin with the Be Well Fab Four! These are the four categories of macronutrients we live by on this program: protein, fat, fiber, and greens. Remember the chart on page 63? These food groups were chosen for a reason.

PROTEIN is the building block of your muscles and other cells. Among other things, protein:

- signals to your brain that you're full. Protein increases production of GLP-1 (your "full" hormone), contributes to satiety due to its interaction with CCK (one of your "satiety" hormones), increases PYY (your "control" hormone), and releases dopamine (your "reward" hormone). (Also, a *lack* of protein increases NPY and "stimulates" your craving for more carbohydrates.)

- contains B vitamins and minerals that help with overall food absorption.
- is a source of amino acids, which are the building blocks of all proteins, including collagen.

FAT is necessary for brain functioning, hormonal production and balance, and cell development and growth. Specifically, essential fatty acids (omega-3 and omega-6 in proper proportions) are critical for managing the hormones that regulate temperature, moods, and digestion. Among other things, fat:

- increases satiety (through leptin and CCK).
- reduces fasting insulin levels.
- makes us feel calmer and more relaxed.
- slows digestion.
- curbs cravings.
- maximizes loss of stored body fat (ketosis).
- hydrates cells.

Some of the go-to sources of "good" fat include avocados, fatty fish (such as salmon, trout, mackerel, sardines, and herring), olive oil, coconut and coconut oil, nuts, and chia seeds. In chapters 7 and 8, I'll show you how to "sneak" these rich sources of fats into your Fab Four Smoothie and Fab Four Roadie, my version of a smoothie that you can take when you're on the go or before a dinner, wedding, bridal shower, birthday, or Super Bowl party when you know your food options might be limited and/or only deep-fried. You'll learn more about this super-fun tool in chapter 8.

FIBER moves food through our digestive system. It's found in nonstarchy carbohydrates such as vegetables, seeds, nuts, and fruits. It's an absolutely necessary part of gut health and regular digestion. Fiber:

- provides food for good bacteria in the gut, which helps keep you regular.
- helps the body produce butyrate, a short-chain fatty acid ("superfat" for the gut) that prevents cancer and has anti-inflammatory properties.
- removes toxins from the body.
- slows absorption of glucose.

In chapter 6, you will learn all about how fiber can be added to your meals, whether on the go or at home.

GREENS (aka: vegetables deep in color), along with being a source of fiber, are nature's way of providing us with the vitamins, minerals, and antioxidants that prevent premature aging, strengthen our immune systems so we can resist disease and illness, and protect our overall health and physical and mental well-being. Diets that are loaded with processed foods don't deliver sufficient vitamins and minerals. Supplements are an alternative, but I am a big fan of introducing greens through the foods you eat. Here's what they do:

- Produce antioxidants that repair cell damage from the environment.
- Serve as anti-inflammatory, anticancer, and detoxification agents.
- Provide naturally occurring resistant starch that feeds gut microbiota.
- Contain the sugar sulfoquinovose that feeds gut microbiota.
- Replace vitamins and minerals.
- Offer medicinal properties for healing.
- Provide phytonutrients and phytochemicals.

PHYTONUTRIENTS

- Beta-carotene: An orange carotenoid found in various vegetables.
- Curcumin: The primary polyphenol in turmeric root.
- Epigallocatechin-3-gallate (EGCG): A green tea extract; abundant in matcha.

- Ellagic acid: Found in berries; may slow the growth of cancer cells and help your liver neutralize cancer-causing chemicals.

- Hesperidin: In citrus fruits such as oranges and lemons; has antioxidant and anti-inflammatory properties.

- Lutein: Found in broccoli, spinach, kale, zucchini, and squash.

- Lycopene: A red carotenoid found in watermelon, pink grapefruit, tomatoes, and pomegranate extracts.

- Luteolin: A flavonoid found in peppers and various green vegetables.

- Piperine: A phytochemical found in black pepper (increases curcumin).

- Quercetin: A well-studied type of flavonol found in berries, apples, kale, and onions.

- Resveratrol: A phytochemical found in grapes, peanuts, and wine.

- Sulforaphane: A sulfurous phytochemical found in cruciferous vegetables that increases enzymes that can deactivate free radicals and carcinogens.

The Fab Four Smoothie and Fab Four are the keys to balanced blood sugar. This scientifically supported, simple-to-put-together formula for meals or a meal replacement smoothie will accomplish all that you want:

- Blood sugar balance.
- Increased satiety.
- Elongated blood sugar curve.
- Insulin sensitivity.

The result? You'll feel energetic yet calm, satisfied and not hungry, and connected to your body on a whole new level. My guess is that you've probably never enjoyed the benefits of putting these feelings together, because either you don't eat to satiety or you listen only to how you "feel" about food when you tell yourself, *I feel like having that doughnut.* But I promise when you make these slight changes to what you are eating and choose from the Fab Four (and my Fab Four Smoothies in chapter 7), you will easily cue in to your body's satiety, keep hungry hormones at bay, and learn to eat in a way that helps you either lose weight or maintain your weight.

GO FOR LIGHT STRUCTURE

Though I've provided portion goals for each of the Fab Four, so that you'll know what the "right amount" looks like for each meal, it's really up to you to make the Fab Four your own. The beauty of this light structure is that you decide what to eat for each category. You can be a salmon-salad-with-avocado lover, a lettuce-wrapped-burger babe, or a shrimp-stir-fry dude. All you have to do is get your portions right, so you feel full and satisfied. The power is in **your hands,** and I'm putting it there on purpose—I want you to learn to trust yourself, feel confident in your decisions, and build the lifestyle you want around the foods you love.

That said, I'm going to give you a *ton* of ideas! This chapter is full of simple, delicious, and filling recipes for Fab Four meals that appeal to all different palates and lifestyle preferences. And if cooking isn't your thing, you can use the recipes as a guide to help you get a sense of what to order when you go out. (More on my Meal Prep Hacks in chapter 8.)

One other thing—notice my choice of words up above. I said *meals,* not snacks. Meals are key. Snacking delays the inevitable and, as I mentioned back in chapter 4, can disrupt your digestion process. If you're hungry, eat a real Fab Four meal (with a Fab Four Smoothie as an option). When you turn off your hunger with enough of the right foods, you're learning to reset your body-brain satiety signals. Essentially, you're learning how to eat only when you are really hungry, not when you are in a craving state. There's a big difference.

Before we get to the portion goals and recipes, let me share two quick client stories with you.

Twenty-nine-year-old Aaron, one of my athletes, was constantly hungry and feeling depleted. He was very active and eating his version of clean: three meals and at least two snacks per day, consisting of things like high-protein cereal with yogurt, an apple and almond butter for a snack, a whole wheat sandwich with fruit, a pre-workout energy bar, and then lots of chicken and rice for dinner. We modified his three meals to be Fab Four meals, and immediately those snacks became history. He continued to use a post-strength-training protein shake to support muscle gain, but he didn't need snacks to bridge between meals. Aaron was shocked at the difference in how he felt—full, energized, and mentally sharp.

Kate, thirty-one, had just weaned her eight-month-old son, Oliver, when we had our first call. Her goal was to lose her last fifteen pounds of baby weight. She was finally getting some sleep, being more mobile on her feet, and thinking about getting a trainer. Kate walked me through her typical day: coffee with vanilla coconut milk creamer, a bite of a banana, a handful of Cheerios, a nibble of chicken, a few blueberries, a handful of cheese puffs, a sip from a pear puree pack, an iced vanilla latte in the afternoon, then a couple of chips with salsa as she made dinner. If I were Kate, by four P.M. I would want a ticket to the all-you-can-eat buffet! Can you guess what happened next? Yep, she overate at dinner and even then wasn't totally satisfied until she had her chocolate fix. Kate never quieted her hunger. She stoked it over and over, and it screamed for her to eat. Do you have any idea how common this is?

Kate was frustrated. She couldn't figure out why she couldn't lose weight, because in her mind she was barely eating and her calories weren't excessive. Can you guess? Was it (a) blood sugar imbalance; (b) hunger hormone imbalance; (c) emotional imbalance that included being "hangry," food obsessed, and body bashing; or **(d) all of the above.** Kate didn't need to change her whole life to start seeing big changes. I asked her to make a Fab Four Smoothie for breakfast and then wait to eat a Fab Four lunch. She would aim to have 20 grams of protein, 2 cups of fibrous green vegetables, and a couple of tablespoons of fat. After a few weeks, Kate no longer needed to eat in the afternoon, and within a month, she had lost eighteen pounds and twenty-two inches all over her body!

I will never forget the e-mail I received from Kate after three months of working together:

> I am crying while I write this e-mail. Kelly, you are my angel, I don't know why or how God brought you into my life but my gratitude is hard to put into words. I have been dieting for over fifteen years and I don't want to even think about the moments I've lost so I won't. Today, I am more confident than I have ever been in a body I didn't think I would ever own. But what brings me to tears is that I have never been more myself. I am a better mom, better wife, and better friend. I am present, joyful, and calm. Thank you for teaching me to trust my body again. I love it and it loves me right back.

A lot of people grab a latte, energy bar, juice, muffin, or 100-calorie pack of something without reviewing the macronutrient content and thinking about what it will do to their hunger. The answer is, not much. Snacking isn't eating to satiety. But remember, when you begin each day with a Fab Four Smoothie or a Fab Four meal, you set yourself up to elongate your blood sugar curve and increase your sense of fullness for up to six hours. And the same goes for lunch. That's a lot of time to be burning calories and helping you lose

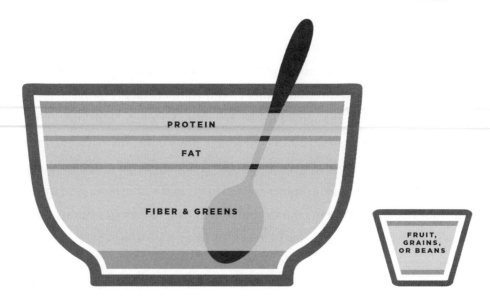

weight! Of course, it does more than that, too. By eating fiber-rich vegetables, you slowly release insulin (instead of asking your pancreas to overdo it) and keep NPY (a carbohydrate-craving hormone) at bay. You give your body the precursors to make the happy hormones—dopamine, norepinephrine, and serotonin. It's not an accident that I sit down to complete meals with every Fab Four component.

FAB FOUR PORTION GOALS

How should your Fab Four be portioned at every meal? Use these guidelines for quantities and review the lists that follow to see what falls into the Fab Four categories:

- Protein: 4 to 6 ounces for women; 6 to 8 ounces for men.
- Fat: 2 tablespoons.
- Fiber and greens: 2 to 4 cups fibrous green vegetables.
- Fruit: $\frac{1}{2}$ cup maximum. It's best to have it in the morning (preferably in your Fab Four Smoothie), so your body has a chance to metabolize it in the liver and the space to store it. Snack or dessert is okay, too, but not all three.
- No more than one serving of a starchy carbohydrate per meal (such as 1 tortilla or $\frac{1}{4}$ to $\frac{1}{2}$ cup gluten-free grain).
- Reduce dairy (such as yogurt or a hard cheese) to 1 to 2 servings per week or less.

YOUR FAB FOUR RECIPES

Most of these recipes take under twenty minutes to prepare and require minimal equipment. My go-to kitchen tools include a food processor, a high-speed blender, a zoodler, a meat thermometer, and a stainless-steel skillet. Since ovens vary, I depend exclusively on my meat thermometer to indicate the doneness of meat.

LEMON-GARLIC ROAST CHICKEN

*This whole roast chicken is great with a side of asparagus, broccolini,
or cauliflower mash. It's an easy and delicious comfort food that's perfect for
a night at home or when you have friends over.*

Makes 2 to 4 servings, depending on the size of the bird

1 tablespoon dried rosemary
1 tablespoon dried thyme
1 tablespoon dried oregano
1 tablespoon sea salt
1 tablespoon olive oil
1 (3-pound) whole chicken
2 lemons, halved
1 garlic head

1. Preheat the oven to 375°F.
2. In a small bowl, combine the rosemary, thyme, oregano, salt, and olive oil.
3. Remove any giblets from inside the chicken and pat it dry with paper towels. Set it in a shallow roasting pan and coat the chicken with the seasoning mix.
4. Stuff 2 lemon halves into the cavity of the chicken and place the other 2 in the pan.
5. Slice the top off the garlic head to make the cloves visible and set it in the cavity of the chicken, cloves out.
6. Bake the chicken for 60 to 75 minutes, until an instant-read thermometer inserted into the breast without touching the bone registers an internal temperature of 170°F.
7. Let the chicken rest for 5 to 10 minutes, then slice and serve.

BROCCOLINI BEEF BOWL

It doesn't get much easier than this, and the taste is sure to satisfy your craving for Asian takeout! This meal was made in under ten minutes, and the minced garlic and ginger came from jars. (Yep, I admit it.)

Makes 2 servings

8 to 10 broccolini stalks, halved crosswise
6 tablespoons coconut aminos
1 tablespoon minced fresh ginger
1 tablespoon minced garlic
1 tablespoon red pepper flakes
2 tablespoons coconut oil
Pink Himalayan salt or sea salt
2 (4- to 6-ounce) grass-finished strip loin steaks, thinly sliced across the grain
Organic stevia drops
Minced fresh chives, for garnish
Sesame seeds, for garnish
Hot sauce

1. Bring 2 inches of water to a simmer in a saucepan over medium heat. Add the broccolini and cook for 4 minutes, or until tender. Drain and set aside.
2. Make your sauce! In a medium bowl, whisk together the coconut aminos, ginger, garlic, and red pepper flakes.
3. In the same saucepan, heat the coconut oil over high heat. Lightly salt the beef and add it to the pan. Cook for 2 minutes, then turn the beef and add the sauce. Cook the beef through for about 2 minutes, stir, and add 4 drops of stevia, or to taste (a little goes a long way).
4. Return the broccolini to the pan, and stir to combine and coat.
5. Serve in a bowl garnished with sesame seeds and chives, with hot sauce alongside.

CHICKEN FAB PHO

This recipe calls for a store-bought rotisserie chicken; try to choose one that is organic and not heavily spiced so you can add your own flavor.

Makes 4 servings

1 tablespoon coconut oil

2 tablespoons minced fresh ginger

2 tablespoons minced garlic

2 quarts Chicken Bone Broth (page 107) or chicken stock

2 tablespoons coconut aminos

2 zucchini, zoodled (see Note)

2 summer squash, zoodled (see Note)

4 small bok choy

1/2 cup bean sprouts

1 store-bought rotisserie chicken, meat shredded

Fresh cilantro

Fresh basil

Red pepper flakes

1. In a medium saucepan, heat the oil over medium heat. Add the ginger and garlic and sauté until fragrant, 1 to 2 minutes. Add the broth and coconut aminos, bring to a boil, and cook for 2 to 3 minutes, or until cooked through.

2. In shallow bowls, layer the veggies and top with the shredded chicken. Top with broth.

3. Top with cilantro, basil, and red pepper flakes.

Note: I love my zoodler (also known as a spiralizer), but you can also use a vegetable peeler to make long, flat strips of the vegetables.

BONE BROTH RECIPE

This richly textured, deeply delicious broth is a supreme immune support and overall anti-inflammatory. An elixir you will enjoy!

Makes 1 to 1¹/₂ quarts (serving size: 1 cup)

About 2 pounds grass-finished beef or pasture-raised chicken bones
1 medium organic carrot, peeled and chopped
1 medium organic onion, chopped
1 organic celery stalk, chopped
3 organic garlic cloves, peeled and roughly chopped
1 teaspoon pink Himalayan salt
1 tablespoon organic apple cider vinegar

1. Place the bones, vegetables, and garlic in a 3-quart slow cooker. Fill the cooker to the top with filtered water and add the salt and vinegar.
2. Cook on low for 18 to 24 hours (The more time, the more flavor, so if it tastes good at 18 hours, you're good to go!)
3. Strain the broth through cheesecloth or a fine-mesh strainer and cool.
4. Store in a glass container in the fridge.

SAUCY PALEO MEATBALLS

My vote for a hearty, satisfying meal!

Makes 8 meatballs, for 2 servings

1 pound 100% grass-finished ground beef (or protein of your choice)
1 large egg
$\frac{1}{4}$ cup flax meal
1 garlic clove, minced
1 tablespoon dried oregano
1 tablespoon dried thyme
$1\frac{1}{2}$ teaspoons pink Himalayan salt
$1\frac{1}{2}$ teaspoons onion powder
2 tablespoons fresh minced or dried parsley
1 (16-ounce) jar of your favorite marinara sauce
Grated goat's- or sheep's-milk Parmesan cheese or yogurt, for serving (optional)
Zucchini or squash zoodles (see Note, page 106), for serving

1. Preheat the oven to 350°F.
2. In a large bowl, use your hands (or a wooden spoon) to combine the beef, egg, flax meal, garlic, oregano, thyme, salt, onion powder, and 1 tablespoon of the parsley. The mixture should be smooth, but don't overmix.
3. Form the mixture into meatballs about 1 inch in diameter and place them on an ungreased rimmed baking sheet. Bake for 12 minutes, or until browned and cooked through.
4. Transfer the meatballs to a decorative oven-safe baking dish. Pour the marinara over the meatballs to cover. Bake for 5 minutes to heat and thicken the sauce.
5. Sprinkle Parmesan over the meatballs and garnish with the remaining parsley. Serve warm, with a side of zoodles.

MINI LAMB CHOPS WITH PISTACHIO-MINT PESTO

This dish is great for a casual get-together or a bigger party.
Roasted asparagus is the perfect accompaniment.

Makes 4 servings

LAMB

Leaves from 3 thyme sprigs, chopped
Leaves from 2 rosemary sprigs, chopped
3 garlic cloves, chopped
1 tablespoon pink Himalayan salt
1 tablespoon freshly ground black pepper
1 tablespoon chili powder
4 tablespoons olive oil
Juice from $\frac{1}{2}$ lemon
1 ($1\frac{1}{2}$-pound) rack of lamb (8 ribs)
$\frac{1}{2}$ cup organic red wine
2 cups fresh packed spinach

PESTO

$\frac{1}{2}$ cup packed fresh mint leaves
$\frac{1}{2}$ cup packed fresh spinach
2 garlic cloves
$\frac{1}{3}$ cup shelled unsalted pistachios
$\frac{3}{4}$ cup olive oil
1 teaspoon sea salt

1. Make the lamb: Preheat the oven to 350°F.
2. In a large bowl, combine the thyme, rosemary, garlic, salt, pepper, chili powder, 2 tablespoons of the olive oil, and the lemon juice. Mix well and set aside. *(cont.)*

3. Trim some fat from the rack of lamb and rub it on all sides with the herb mixture.

4. In a large cast-iron pan or other oven-safe skillet, heat the remaining 2 tablespoons oil over medium heat. Add the lamb and sear for 2 minutes per side. Add the wine and place the pan in the oven. Roast the lamb until the internal temperature reaches 145°F (medium-rare), about 10 minutes. Let the lamb rest for a few minutes before slicing into chops.

5. While the lamb is roasting, make the pesto: Combine all the pesto ingredients in high-speed blender or food processor and blend until well combined.

6. Serve the lamb chops with the pesto drizzled on top.

TURKEY-STUFFED DELICATA SQUASH

Want to add to a Thanksgiving feast? Offer to make this delicate dish!

Makes 4 servings

2 (1-pound) delicata squash, sliced lengthwise and seeded
4 tablespoons olive oil
Pink Himalayan salt and freshly ground black pepper
1 cup chopped onion
1 cup chopped celery
2 garlic cloves, minced
1 cup chopped mushrooms
1 pound ground turkey
1 tablespoon organic garlic salt
$^1/_2$ teaspoon smoked paprika
1 teaspoon ground cumin
1 cup chopped kale leaves
2 tablespoons tahini
2 tablespoons minced fresh chives

1. Preheat the oven to 425°F.

2. Rub the squash halves with 2 tablespoons olive oil and season the insides with salt and pepper. Set them cut-side up in a baking dish or rimmed baking sheet and roast for 35 minutes, or until tender.

3. In a large skillet, heat the remaining 2 tablespoons olive oil over medium heat. Add the onion, celery, and garlic and cook until the onion is translucent, 4 to 5 minutes. Add the mushrooms and cook until tender, 2 to 3 minutes. Add the turkey, garlic salt, paprika, and cumin and cook until the turkey is cooked through (usually about 4 to 5 minutes), breaking it up as needed. Add the kale and cook for 1 to 2 minutes, until softened.

4. Take the pan off the heat. Stir in the tahini and season with salt and pepper.

5. Divide the turkey mixture among the squash halves (they should be generously full). Sprinkle with chives and serve a squash half to each person.

BUFFALO CHILI

Yum—perfect for watching the game at home or tailgating.

Makes 8 to 10 servings (1 cup each)

1½ tablespoons olive oil
½ medium white onion
2 celery stalks, diced
1 garlic clove, minced
1 pound ground buffalo meat
2 tablespoons chili powder
1½ teaspoons smoked paprika
½ teaspoon dried oregano
½ teaspoon cayenne
½ teaspoon ground cumin

(cont.)

1 teaspoon pink Himalayan salt

$^1/_2$ teaspoon freshly ground black pepper

1 (28-ounce) can crushed tomatoes

2 cups vegetable broth

1 green bell pepper, chopped

1 tablespoon chopped green onions

Avocado chunks, for serving

1. In a large pot, heat the oil over medium-low heat. Add the onion, celery, and garlic and sauté until the onion is translucent. Add the meat, breaking it up into small pieces with a spoon as it cooks. Stir in the chili powder, paprika, oregano, cayenne, cumin, salt, and black pepper and cook until the meat is evenly browned, about 6 minutes.

2. Add the tomatoes, broth, and bell pepper and stir. Bring to a boil. Reduce the heat to low, cover, and simmer for 20 to 30 minutes to allow the flavors to develop.

3. Serve with avocado chunks alongside, and enjoy!

CHIA FLAX CHICKEN TENDERS

We all love the tasty comfort of a chicken tender. Try this one, with an added bump of fat and fiber—so delicious!

Makes 4 to 6 servings

1 cup potato starch

1 teaspoon pink Himalayan salt

1 teaspoon freshly ground black pepper

2 large eggs

1 cup chia seeds

1 cup flaxseeds

1 cup gluten-free panko bread crumbs (or grain-free flour)

2 teaspoons paprika

2 teaspoons garlic salt

Pinch of chopped fresh parsley

4 to 6 ounces uncooked chicken tenders, pounded to $^1/_2$ inch thick or less

$^1/_4$ cup ghee (clarified butter)

Avocado Hummus (page 125), for serving

1. Preheat the oven to 350°F.

2. Create a breading line. On one plate, combine the potato starch, salt, and pepper. In a shallow bowl, whisk the eggs. On a second plate, combine the chia, flax, bread crumbs, paprika, garlic salt, and parsley.

3. Take each chicken tender through the breading line, first dipping it in the potato starch mixture, then dredging it in the egg mixture to coat completely, letting the excess drip off, then coating it with the chia-flax mixture. Set the pieces on a baking sheet as you finish.

4. In a large sauté pan, melt the ghee over medium heat.

5. Working in batches, set the tenders in the pan and raise the heat to medium-high. Cook the tenders, turning them gently after 2 to 4 minutes, until the crumbs are browned on both sides and the chicken is cooked through. Transfer them to a baking dish or baking sheet as you finish each batch.

6. Transfer the tenders to the oven and bake for 10 to 12 minutes, or until cooked through.

7. Serve with avocado hummus.

AVOCADO CHICKEN SALAD BOAT

A great appetizer or a light yet filling meal!

Makes 4 meal-size servings or appetizers for 12

2 chicken breasts, cooked, cooled, and shredded
2 large avocados, pitted, peeled, and roughly mashed
¼ cup chopped fresh cilantro
¼ cup chopped fresh chives
Juice of 1 lime
1 tablespoon pink Himalayan salt
4 Belgian endive heads, separated into leaves, or 2 cucumbers, halved lengthwise

1. In a large bowl, combine the chicken, avocado, cilantro, and chives and stir until the chicken is well coated with the avocado.
2. Add the lime juice and sprinkle with the salt. Mix to combine.
3. Serve the chicken salad in the endive leaves, or make mini cucumber boats by scooping out the cucumber seeds with the tip of a spoon and spreading the chicken salad inside the cucumber halves.

FAB FOUR FISH POCKETS

*If you tend to stay away from preparing seafood,
start with this easy-to-make recipe.*

Makes 2 servings

4 to 6 ounces fish of choice (salmon, halibut, sole)
1 to 2 cups chopped vegetables of choice (zucchini, summer squash, asparagus, broccolini)

1 tablespoon aromatic of choice (garlic, onion, shallot, chives)

1 tablespoon minced fresh or dried herb of choice (parsley, thyme, sage, herbes de
Provence, cilantro)

1 tablespoon fat of choice (olive oil, melted coconut oil, melted butter)

1. Preheat the oven to 350°F.

2. On a large piece of parchment paper, layer the fish, vegetables, aromatic, and
herbs. Drizzle with the fat.

3. Fold or crimp the parchment paper into a sealed pocket. Bake for 20 minutes,
or until the fish is cooked through. Serve in the paper for extra drama!

SALMON POKE BOWL

I love poke *bowls, and this one is a favorite!*

Makes 2 servings

2 tablespoons coconut aminos

1 teaspoon rice vinegar

1 teaspoon sesame oil

1 teaspoon sesame seeds, plus more for garnish

$^1/_2$ teaspoon red pepper flakes

$^1/_2$ pound sushi-grade salmon, cut into 1-inch cubes

2 or 3 scallions, thinly sliced

1 ripe avocado

4 cups chopped kale leaves

1 cup sliced cucumber

1. In a medium bowl, whisk together the coconut aminos, vinegar, oil, sesame
seeds, and red pepper flakes. Add the salmon and scallions and gently stir to
dress the salmon. Set aside to marinate for 5 minutes. *(cont.)*

2. Meanwhile, pit, peel, and cube the avocado into chunks the size of the salmon. Add to the bowl and mix gently.

3. To serve, divide the kale between two bowls. Top with the *poke* and sliced cucumbers.

BUTTER-LETTUCE-WRAPPED SHRIMP TACOS

The crunch and savory goodness of this dish will make it a weeknight go-to meal.

Makes 2 to 4 servings

1 pound raw wild shrimp, shelled and deveined

1 to 2 tablespoons homemade taco seasoning (see page 183)

$^1/_4$ cup Primal Kitchen mayonnaise (I prefer Primal's mayo because its eggs are pasture-raised and avocado oil contains very little sugar)

Juice of 1 lime

4 cups shredded cabbage (from about $^1/_2$ cabbage)

2 tablespoons avocado oil or other high-smoke-point oil

1 butter lettuce head, leaves separated

1 avocado, pitted, peeled, and cut into small cubes

$^1/_4$ cup chopped fresh cilantro

Lime wedges, for serving

1. In a medium bowl, coat the shrimp with the taco seasoning.

2. In a large bowl, mix the mayonnaise with the lime juice and whisk until thinned. Add the cabbage and mix to coat.

3. In a large skillet, heat the oil over medium heat. Add the shrimp and cook until pink and cooked through, 4 to 5 minutes.

4. Place the lettuce leaves on a plate and use them as taco "shells," layering in the shrimp, slaw, avocado, and cilantro. Squeeze the lime wedges on top and serve.

LEMON-DILL ROASTED SALMON OVER ARUGULA AND MÂCHE

An elegant meal for special guests or a romantic dinner for two, this salmon dish is loaded with nutrition and flavor.

Makes 2 servings

2 (4-ounce) salmon fillets, skin removed
2 tablespoons olive oil
Pink Himalayan salt
$^1/_2$ lemon, thinly sliced
Juice of $^1/_2$ lemon
$^1/_4$ cup extra-virgin olive oil
2 cups arugula leaves
2 cups mâche leaves
Fresh dill, for garnish

1. Preheat the oven to 350°F. Line a baking sheet with aluminum foil.
2. Rub each salmon fillet with 1 tablespoon olive oil and season with salt. Place the salmon on the prepared baking sheet. Top each fillet with a few lemon slices and bake until cooked to your liking, about 20 minutes.
3. In a salad bowl, whisk together the lemon juice and the extra-virgin olive oil.
4. Add the arugula and mâche to the bowl with the dressing and toss to coat.
5. Divide the salad between two serving plates. Top each with a salmon fillet and garnish with dill.

SUMMER CEVICHE JICAMA TACOS

Crunchy goodness wrapped in deliciousness!

Makes 4 servings

1 large jicama, peeled
1 pound medium or large raw shrimp, peeled, deveined, and chopped into small pieces
1 cup fresh lime juice (from about 8 limes)
1 cup fresh lemon juice (from 6 to 8 lemons)
$^1/_4$ cup finely diced mango
1 cup finely diced Persian cucumber
1 cup finely diced red bell pepper
$^1/_2$ cup chopped fresh cilantro, plus more for serving
$^1/_4$ cup finely diced red onion
3 tablespoons minced serrano pepper
1 avocado, pitted, peeled, and diced
Pink Himalayan salt
Lime wedges, for serving

1. Use a mandoline to cut the jicama into $^1/_8$-inch-thick round slices (these will be your taco "shells") and place them in a large bowl of water with a pinch of salt. Let sit for 20 minutes to 1 hour to remove excess starch and make the jicama malleable.

2. Meanwhile, place the shrimp in a large bowl. Add $^1/_2$ cup of the lime juice and $^1/_2$ cup of the lemon juice. Let stand so the shrimp can "cook" in the juice, about 15 minutes, or until the shrimp are pink and opaque.

3. In a separate large bowl, combine the remaining $^1/_2$ cup lime juice and $^1/_2$ cup lemon juice, the mango, cucumber, bell pepper, cilantro, onion, and serrano pepper and mix well. Transfer the vegetable mixture to the bowl with the shrimp and mix well to incorporate. Season with salt and mix well.

4. Add the avocado cubes to the ceviche and garnish with cilantro just before serving.

5. Fill your jicama taco shells with ceviche and finish with a squeeze of lime and a pinch of salt.

GRAPEFRUIT SALMON CRUDO

This dish is an easy one to make on the run. Head to your local grocery store or fish purveyor to pick up some sushi-grade salmon, add the grapefruit, avocado, and lemon juice, and you have an instant meal or hearty appetizer!

Makes 2 servings

$1/2$ pound sushi-grade salmon, thinly sliced
1 avocado, pitted, peeled, and cut into small cubes
1 pink grapefruit, suprêmed (see Note)
1 red radish, thinly sliced
2 tablespoons avocado oil
1 tablespoon fresh grapefruit juice
1 tablespoon lemon juice
Pink Himalayan salt and cracked black pepper

1. On two serving plates, layer the salmon, avocado, grapefruit suprêmes, and radish, dividing them evenly.

2. In a small bowl, whisk together the oil, grapefruit juice, and lemon juice and season with salt and pepper.

3. Drizzle the dressing over the crudo and serve.

Note: To suprême a grapefruit (or any citrus), cut a slice from one end of the grapefruit so it will stand flat on your cutting board. With a sharp knife, cut the peel and white pith away, leaving as much fruit behind as you can. Working over a bowl, cut along the grapefruit segments to release them from the membrane, letting them drop into the bowl as you go. You can use the juice that collects in the bowl for the crudo dressing!

SPICY SALMON NORI BURRITO

The spice gives the salmon an extra kick!

Makes 2 servings

¹/₄ cup Primal Kitchen mayonnaise

1 to 2 tablespoons Organicville gluten-free Sky Valley Sriracha Sauce (another super clean brand!)

1 (6-ounce) can wild salmon, drained

1 (10-sheet) package 7 × 8-inch dried nori wraps

1 cup cooked quinoa or brown rice (optional)

1 cup mixed greens

1 tablespoon olive oil

1¹/₂ teaspoons rice vinegar

1 avocado, pitted, peeled, and thinly sliced

¹/₂ cup sliced peeled cucumber

¹/₂ cup shredded carrot

1 tablespoon sesame seeds

¹/₄ cup coconut aminos

1. Preheat the oven to 350°F. Line a baking sheet with parchment paper.

2. In a medium bowl, combine the mayo and sriracha. Add the salmon and mix gently with a fork.

3. Place 2 nori sheets on the prepared baking sheet and top each with ¹/₂ cup of the quinoa (if using) and half the salmon salad. Warm the wraps in the oven for 3 to 5 minutes, until the nori is malleable (if the quinoa is warm, you won't need to use the oven).

4. In a medium bowl, dress the greens with the oil and vinegar. Toss to coat.

5. Layer the nori wraps with the avocado, cucumber, carrot, and mixed greens. Roll each into a burrito (ends tucked in) and cut in half. Garnish with the sesame seeds and serve with coconut aminos for dipping.

FRENCH SALMON SALAD

If you're looking for a dish that can work as lunch or dinner, this salad does the trick.

Makes 1 or 2 servings

1 (6-ounce) can wild salmon, drained
1 tablespoon Primal Kitchen mayonnaise
1 tablespoon whole-grain Dijon mustard
4 tablespoons olive oil
1 tablespoon capers
1 tablespoon chopped shallot
1 tablespoon chopped fresh dill
1 tablespoon champagne vinegar
Pink Himalayan salt and freshly ground black pepper
1 bag organic salad greens

1. In a medium bowl, break up the salmon with a fork. Add the mayo, mustard, 1 tablespoon of the oil, the capers, shallot, and dill and mix carefully.
2. In a salad bowl, whisk together the vinegar and remaining 3 tablespoons oil until emulsified. Season with salt and pepper. Add the salad greens and toss to coat in the dressing.
3. Divide the greens between plates and top with the salmon salad or leave them in the bowl if you're keeping this one all to yourself!

ANTI-INFLAMMATORY DETOX SALAD

This dish may not have a sexy name, but it works!

Makes 2 servings

2 tablespoons apple cider vinegar

¼ cup olive oil

½ teaspoon ground turmeric

Squeeze of fresh lemon juice

1 teaspoon honey

4 cups mixed baby spinach and kale

1 or 2 Persian cucumbers, sliced

6 to 8 asparagus stalks, trimmed and cut into 1-inch pieces

½ cup microgreens

1 avocado, pitted, peeled, and cut into small cubes

2 tablespoons chopped fresh parsley

2 tablespoons chopped fresh cilantro

2 tablespoons chopped fresh dill

1. In a salad bowl, whisk together the dressing ingredients.

2. Add the salad ingredients and toss to coat with the dressing.

3. Divide the salad between two plates and serve.

4. Option to top with protein such as 4 ounces of chicken, salmon, or shrimp.

CHICKEN KALE COBB SNOB SALAD

Yum—this recipe combines some of my favorite building blocks,
resulting in a tasty yet super nutritious meal on wheels.

Makes 2 servings

DRESSING

$\frac{1}{2}$ cup extra-virgin olive oil

$\frac{1}{4}$ cup red wine vinegar

Juice of $\frac{1}{2}$ lemon

1 tablespoon gluten-free Worcestershire sauce

1 teaspoon Dijon mustard

Pink Himalayan salt and freshly ground black pepper

SALAD

4 cups chopped kale

1 cooked organic chicken breast, chopped

2 hard-boiled eggs, sliced

2 organic nitrate-free bacon slices, cooked and crumbled

$\frac{1}{4}$ cup chopped cashews

$\frac{1}{4}$ cup shredded carrot (optional)

$\frac{1}{4}$ cup shredded red cabbage (optional)

$\frac{1}{4}$ cup halved cherry tomatoes

1. In a salad bowl, whisk together the dressing ingredients.

2. Add the salad ingredients and toss to coat with the dressing.

3. Divide the salad between two plates and serve.

THAI PEANUT SLAW

When you're looking for something a little different, try this
satisfying slaw that can be a side dish or main course.

Makes 8 servings (1 cup each)

PEANUT DRESSING
6 tablespoons raw almond or peanut butter
2 tablespoons coconut aminos
2 tablespoons rice vinegar
2 tablespoons untoasted sesame oil
2 teaspoons fresh lime juice
2 garlic cloves, crushed
Red pepper flakes

SLAW
$\frac{1}{2}$ head red cabbage
$\frac{1}{2}$ head Napa cabbage
4 or 5 carrots
1 jalapeño, minced (optional)
1 cup unsalted peanuts

1. Make the dressing: In a high-speed blender or food processor, combine all the dressing ingredients and blend until smooth. Pour into a small bowl and set aside.
2. Place the red cabbage in high-powered blender or food processor and blend using the slicer blade.
3. Add the Napa cabbage and blend with the slicer blade.
4. Then add the carrots, using the shredder blade.
5. In a large mixing bowl, combine the shredded cabbage and carrots mixture, and add minced jalapeño to your desired heat. Stir in the dressing, top with peanuts, and serve.

HOMEMADE HUMMUS

It is so easy to make your own hummus. This basic recipe can be tweaked to use whatever flavor you're looking for—cilantro, basil, sriracha, you name it.

Makes 4 to 5 cups

1 (15-ounce) can garbanzo beans (chickpeas), drained and rinsed
1 garlic clove, minced
Juice of ½ lemon
Pink Himalayan salt
⅛ to ¼ cup olive oil

> In a blender, combine the beans, garlic, lemon juice, and salt to taste and blend for 2 to 3 minutes. With the motor running, drizzle in the olive oil, using more or less to reach your desired consistency.

AVOCADO HUMMUS

This is a versatile side that can work as a dip with crunchy veggies or as a tasty fat sauce, or as a good bridge snack.

Makes 4 to 5 cups

3 avocados, pitted and peeled
1 to 2 tablespoons tahini
1 to 2 garlic cloves
Squeeze of fresh lemon juice
Extra-virgin olive oil
Hemp hearts and sesame seeds, for serving

> In a high-speed blender or food processor, combine the avocados, tahini, garlic, and lemon juice. Add a drizzle of olive oil and blend fast. Top with a mix of hemp hearts and sesame seeds.

125

CHIMICHURRI SAUCE

One of my favorite fat sauces, chimichurri hails from Argentina, but I use it to give some zest to all sorts of dishes.

Makes ¹/₂ cup

2 cups chopped fresh parsley (I prefer leaves only, but it's up to you!)
1 garlic clove
¹/₄ cup olive oil
1 tablespoon red pepper flakes
2 tablespoons fresh oregano
Squeeze of fresh lemon juice
Walnuts (optional)

In a high-speed blender or food processor, combine all the ingredients and blend until smooth. If you want a thicker sauce, add a few walnuts and blend again until smooth.

SWEET-AND-SALTY WALNUT BUTTER

Use a version of this recipe to make any type of butter you love! Consider mixing two types of nuts, such as walnuts and cashews.

Makes 1 cup

1 cup raw walnuts, frozen for 30 minutes (see Note)
2 teaspoons raw honey
2 teaspoons sea salt

1. In a food processor, pulse the nuts and 1 teaspoon honey until a ball of butter forms. Add 1 teaspoon salt and process to combine.

2. Scoop the mixture into a bowl and stir in the remaining 1 teaspoon honey and 1 teaspoon salt by hand.

Note: Using frozen nuts keeps them from heating while processing, which preserves their anti-inflammatory oils.

CILANTRO PESTO

This is another fat sauce and dip you can serve with veggies.

Makes 2 cups

3 cups chopped fresh cilantro
3 tablespoons minced and seeded jalapeño (from 1 to 2 medium)
1 garlic clove
1 cup raw pistachios
1 cup extra-virgin olive oil
Juice of 1 lime
Pink Himalayan salt

In a food processor, combine all the ingredients and pulse until the desired texture is reached.

FAB FOUR VINAIGRETTE

A tasty dressing fit for all salads, greens, and crunchy veggies.
You can store this dressing in the fridge for up to a week.

Makes 1^1/$_2$ cups

^{1}/$_4$ cup champagne vinegar (red wine vinegar and apple cider vinegar work well, too)
1 tablespoon Dijon mustard
1 tablespoon fresh lemon juice
1 tablespoon minced garlic
1 teaspoon pink Himalayan salt
1 cup extra-virgin olive oil

Blender Bottle Directions

1. Put all the ingredients in a blender bottle and shake until the dressing emulsifies completely.
2. Pull out of the fridge 30 minutes before use to let the oil liquefy.
3. Shake and use to dress your salad.

Whisk Directions

1. In a medium bowl, whisk together the vinegar, mustard, lemon juice, garlic, and salt until the salt has dissolved.
2. While whisking, slowly add the oil and whisk until emulsified.

DILL RANCH DRESSING

For salad or for dipping chicken fingers or your fave crunchy veggies.

Makes 1¹/₂ cups

3 tablespoons coconut milk (regular or light)
3 tablespoons Primal Kitchen mayonnaise
2 tablespoons red wine vinegar
1 tablespoon fresh lemon juice
2 tablespoons extra-virgin olive oil
1 tablespoon organic garlic salt
¹/₄ cup finely chopped fresh parsley
¹/₄ cup finely chopped dill
2 tablespoons minced fresh chives

In a medium bowl, whisk together the coconut milk, mayonnaise, vinegar, lemon juice, olive oil, and garlic salt. Add the parsley, dill, and chives and mix gently.

LEMON AIOLI

A versatile sauce that pairs with the roasted asparagus dish and others.
Try it with any grilled seafood or chicken!

Makes 1¹/₄ cups

2 garlic cloves, minced
1 cup Primal Kitchen mayonnaise
2 tablespoons fresh lemon juice
1 tablespoon grated lemon zest
¹/₂ teaspoon pink Himalayan salt

In a blender, combine all the ingredients and blend until smooth.

LEMON VINAIGRETTE

This lovely and light dressing can brighten salads and poultry.

Makes 1¹/₂ cups

Juice of 1 lemon
1 garlic clove, minced
Pinch of Maldon sea salt
³/₄ cup extra-virgin olive oil

In a small bowl, whisk together the lemon juice, garlic, and salt. While whisking, drizzle in the olive oil and whisk until emulsified.

ROASTED ASPARAGUS WITH LEMON AIOLI AND WALNUT PICCATA

I love this side dish, especially when fresh organic asparagus is in season in the spring!

Makes 4 servings

1 tablespoon olive oil
1 pound asparagus, trimmed
Lemon Aioli (page 129)
1 cup grated or chopped walnuts

1. In a large skillet, heat the oil over medium heat. Add the asparagus and cook, stirring occasionally, for 7 to 10 minutes, until the asparagus blister.
2. Plate the asparagus and top with the lemon aioli and walnuts.

BROCCOLINI WITH HAZELNUTS

Give your broccolini some added crunch and savory sweetness.

Makes 4 servings

1 or 2 bunches organic broccolini
1 to 2 tablespoons avocado oil
¹/₂ cup whole unsalted hazelnuts
1 teaspoon pink Himalayan salt, or to taste

1. In a large skillet, heat the oil over medium heat. Add the broccolini and cook, stirring, for 6 to 8 minutes, or until tender.
2. In a small dry skillet, toast the hazelnuts over medium heat until lightly browned, 1 to 2 minutes, stirring often so that they don't burn.
3. Toss the hazelnuts with the broccolini, season with salt, and serve.

CAULIFLOWER AVOCADO MICROGREEN SALAD

This hearty salad is a fan favorite—enjoy! Arugula microgreens are absolutely packed with nutrition.

Makes 4 servings

4 cups mixed organic purple and orange cauliflower florets
1 to 2 tablespoons ghee (clarified butter) or coconut oil, melted
2 cups arugula microgreens
1 avocado, pitted, peeled, and diced

1. Preheat the oven to 400°F.
2. In a large bowl, toss the cauliflower with the melted ghee to coat well.   *(cont.)*

3. Spread the cauliflower on a rimmed baking sheet and roast for 20 to 30 minutes, stirring occasionally, until tender and caramelized.

4. To serve, spread the microgreens on a plate. Top with the cauliflower and diced avocado.

ROASTED GARLIC CASHEW CREAM SAUCE

This fat sauce dresses up veggies and fish. Tangy and terrific!

Makes 2 cups

2 cups organic whole cashews
1 garlic head
1 tablespoon olive oil
1 teaspoon pink Himalayan salt

1. In a medium bowl, cover the cashews with water and let them soak for 2 hours. Drain and rinse.

2. Preheat the oven to 400°F.

3. Break the garlic head into individual cloves (leave the skins on) and place them on a piece of aluminum foil. Top with the olive oil and seal the foil to enclose the garlic. Roast for 30 minutes, or until the garlic is soft.

4. Press the garlic out of the skins into a food processor or high-speed blender. Add the cashews and 1 cup water and blend until smooth. Stir in the salt.

ROASTED VEGETABLE CHICKPEA CURRY BOWL

Beans are an inexpensive and filling plant-based protein.
They are one of the ten pantry staples I always have on hand, and can
be used to quickly upgrade a veggie side to a hearty main.

Makes 2 servings

4 cups mixed 1-inch-cubed eggplant and zucchini and small broccoli florets
2 tablespoons coconut oil, melted, plus 1 tablespoon
1 cup canned or cooked chickpeas, drained and rinsed
1/4 cup chopped onion
1 (13.5-ounce) can coconut milk (regular or light)
3 tablespoons curry powder
1/2 teaspoon pink Himalayan salt
1 date, sliced
2 lemon slices
Cilantro sprigs, for garnish

1. Preheat the oven to 425°F.
2. Toss the vegetables in the melted coconut oil and spread them on a rimmed baking sheet. Roast for 10 minutes, or until golden brown.
3. Turn the veggies over with a spatula and add the chickpeas to the baking sheet. Roast for 10 minutes.
4. Meanwhile, in a large saucepan, heat the remaining 1 tablespoon coconut oil over medium heat. Add the onion and cook, stirring, until tender and translucent. Add the coconut milk, curry, and salt. Whisk and bring to a rolling boil.
5. Add the roasted vegetables and chickpeas to the curry sauce and stir to coat and combine.
6. Serve garnished with the sliced date, lemon, and cilantro.

FREEZER FUDGE

Pop a cube when you need a treat to soothe your sweet tooth.

Makes as many as will fit in your ice cube tray.

1 cup coconut oil
$^1/_4$ cup organic unsweetened cocoa powder
8 to 10 drops liquid stevia
$^1/_4$ to $^1/_2$ cup almond butter (optional)
Maldon sea salt or pink Himalayan salt (optional)

1. Melt the coconut oil in microwave-safe glass bowl.
2. Whisk in the cocoa powder and stevia. Add almond butter to taste if you want a thicker consistency.
3. Divide the mixture among the wells of an ice cube tray (do not fill to the top) and sprinkle with salt, if desired.
4. Freeze for 20 minutes, then turn out of the ice cube tray and store in an airtight container in the fridge for an after-dinner treat!

7

THE FAB FOUR SMOOTHIE: YOUR SECRET WEAPON

THERE'S A SMOOTHIE CRAZE now, and every nutritionist I know seems to have created a smoothie that bursts with flavor and healthy benefits. That's all great. But I didn't create the Fab Four Smoothie to ride the trend with everyone else.

My formula grew organically from my practice, as many of my clients didn't have time to cook a Fab Four breakfast every day. In order to balance their blood sugar and prime their body chemistry and metabolism for the rest of the day, I needed a way to get them the Fab Four in under sixty seconds of prep time—no joke! And I wanted to do it in a tasty, delicious, and satisfying way. (I've tried my fair share of diet shakes in the past, and know how bland and "chalky" they can be.) So, with my science coat and chef hat on, I went to work. What evolved was the Be Well Smoothie—a Fab Four meal that is easy to make in more than *forty* amazing flavors and recipes! Just to name a few of the delicious recipes that follow:

- **SWEET:** Salted Caramel, Snickerdoodle, Apple Pie, Blueberry Muffin, Banana Bread, Lemon Cookie, and Chocolate Cherry
- **CHILL:** Mint Chip, Watermelon Mint, Spa Day, and Strawberry Basil
- **THROWBACKS:** PB&J, Oatmeal Raisin, and Pumpkin Pie
- **FUN:** Mojito, Mango Kale Madness, and Peaches and Greens
- **GREEN:** Mean Matcha, Berry Green, Avocado Green Dream, Açai Green, and Green Apple

The Fab Four Smoothie will be your secret weapon!

My Fab Four Smoothie is a formula based on the same combination of the Fab Four. It is designed to create a blood-sugar-balancing, meal replacement shake in any flavor, with enough protein, fat, fiber, and greens to keep you full for up to six hours. By beginning the day with one of my many smoothie recipes, you set yourself up for balanced blood sugar, a feeling of satiety, and a body chemistry that prompts weight loss through the burning of stored fat. You prime your chemistry with breakfast and set yourself up for success. Imagine that—a day of no cravings, no mood or energy swings. You will feel clearheaded, energetic, and light on your feet. You won't be counting the hours until lunch or dinner or falling victim to sugary temptations.

Here's the formula:

Protein (20 grams minimum)

+ fiber (10 grams or 1 to 2 tablespoons)

+ fat (1 to 2 tablespoons)

+ handful of greens

+ $\frac{1}{4}$ cup fruit

+ superfoods

+ liquid

= Satiety and elongated blood sugar curve

But before we break out the blender, there are a few things you should know. It's important to have the right mind-set regarding smoothies. They're not about starving yourself or trying to survive only on liquids. They're not a diet unto themselves, and they're not the beginning stage of a cleanse. Like the rest of my plan, the Fab Four Smoothie is rooted in the science of blood sugar balance and is formulated to deliver the macronutrients (protein, fat, fiber, and greens) your body needs to be healthy, function properly, and feel sated. It's a tool to use to get you going in the morning, plan ahead before a party, recalibrate if you're out of balance, and fill in for a meal if you're not very hungry. It's *not* a blanket substitute for regular food and Fab Four meals.

There are a lot of other smoothies out there. Beware! Many of the smoothies found at juice shops and grocery smoothie bars and on the Internet are loaded with way, way too much sugar—specifically, fructose from excessive amounts of fruit, agave, dates, and fruit juice. Can you guess what happens when you take in all those simple carbohydrates? Your blood sugar skyrockets. It's like a tall stack of pancakes in a glass. Many of my Fab Four Smoothie recipes include fruit, but in a measured way ($\frac{1}{4}$ to $\frac{1}{2}$ cup) that won't buy you a ticket for the roller coaster. They can also be made fruit-free, depending on your goals and preference.

If you have enough protein, fat, and fiber at each meal, you can elongate your blood sugar curve, which means you will have the energy to maintain a four- to six-hour window between meals. This window will allow your body to properly digest your food, surge with human growth hormone and testosterone to burn fat, calm insulin levels (which slow fat burning), and make you feel more relaxed. The Fab Four Smoothie is designed to make it all possible.

Depending on your previous eating habits (let's say you ate lots of starchy carbohydrates, sugar, or fruit), it might take a little more to hold you over till lunch. I counsel my clients to start with the base formula and see how long their sense of fullness lasts. If they get hungry after just three hours, it's a sign they need to add an extra tablespoon of fiber the next day. If they still get hungry at three and half hours, I tell them to add an extra tablespoon of fat the next day. If the added fiber and fat still don't get them all the way to lunch, then I suggest upping their protein from 20 grams to 30 grams. The more you are tuned into your body and how you are feeling, the more precisely you can create a smoothie that gives you that magic four- to six-hour window of satisfaction.

Think of the Fab Four Smoothie as a formula for creating a custom drink. Find something you like in each category and combine it in the right proportions for something that's personalized and good for you. Here's the breakdown of the formula for a single Fab Four Smoothie:

For **protein,** look for a clean-sprouted vegetarian protein or grass-fed whey.
For **fiber,** use raw fiber powder or chia seeds, flaxseeds, acacia fiber, or even avocado, which is both a fat and a fiber.
Greens can be anything green and/or leafy: kale, spinach, basil, parsley, cucumber . . .
Fruit or high-fructose vegetables can be whatever you like—berries, banana, mango, peach, carrot. Just be sure not to overdo it ($^1/_4$ to $^1/_2$ cup). Frozen fruits are great if you like a thicker smoothie.

Fats can be coconut oil, avocado, nut butter, or walnuts, or try MCT (medium-chain triglyceride) oil.

Liquids can be water, almond milk, coconut water (no added sugar), cashew milk, cold-pressed green juice, walnut milk, or hemp milk. I do *not* recommend dairy (cow milk). **If you go with coconut water or cold-pressed green juice, don't add fruit!**

Last but not least, any **superfood** or additives you want (see the recipes and/or packaging for serving sizes). Here are some of my favorites:

- **ADAPTOGENS:** ashwagandha or Rhodiola, to combat stress and high cortisol
- **RESISTANT STARCH:** potato starch, a prebiotic (see below)
- **SUPER POWDERS:** greens, ginger, turmeric
- **NUTRITIONAL TOPPINGS:** chia seeds, sunflower seeds, coconut flakes, cacao nibs, bee pollen, or sea salt. Use them for flavor or for your particular health goals.

Now, to the recipes!

INTRODUCING UNMODIFIED POTATO STARCH!

A note on introducing unmodified potato starch!

You may recall that resistant starch acts as a strong prebiotic fiber and is found in foods such as sunchokes. When you use the powdered form as a supplement, make sure you start slowly with only a small amount, about 1/4 teaspoon. This wonderful gut builder can give off a lot of gas! You never want to use more than a teaspoon.

THE FAB FOUR SMOOTHIE RECIPES

All the smoothie recipes are designed to serve one person, but you can always double or triple a batch if you are feeding more than one. You can use any kind of high-speed blender. The more power, the smoother and well blended the finish; however, consistency is often just a matter of taste. Keep in mind that the ingredients and measurements are tied to the Fab Four formula, but you might need more or less of any one of the macronutrients—protein, fiber, or fat—depending on your specific goals and how you feel.

Your Fab Four Smoothie Ingredients List

Here's a handy list of the ingredients you will be needing to make your Fab Four Smoothies.

Bulk-buy nonperishables

Protein (20 grams to 30 grams per serving, usually 2 scoops):

- Chocolate protein powder
- Vanilla protein powder
- Plain protein powder
- Collagen protein powder

Fat (1 to 2 tablespoons):

- MCT oil
- Coconut oil
- Olive oil
- Nut butters (unopened; store opened nut butters in the fridge and keep an eye on their expiration date)

- Nuts: raw almonds, cashews, pecans, walnuts, macadamia nuts, Brazil nuts, pistachios
- Seeds: sesame seeds, hemp seeds, sunflower seeds

Fiber (1 to 2 tablespoons):

- Acacia fiber
- Raw fiber powder
- Chia seeds
- Flaxseeds

Greens powder (1 to 2 tablespoons—make sure you check the serving size on the label):

- Greens powder
- Matcha powder

Superfoods (1 teaspoon):

- Hemp hearts
- Cacao nibs
- Adaptogens: ashwagandha, Rhodiola, reishi
- Superfoods: açai powder, maca

Liquid:

- Almond milk (unopened, in a carton)
- Coconut milk (unopened, in a carton; if canned, BPA-free)
- Tea bags: green, hibiscus, mint, lavender, ginger

Perishables

Fridge:

- Fresh almond butter (organic)
- Peanut butter (organic)
- Sunflower butter (organic)

- Walnut butter (organic)
- Avocados
- Cashew butter (organic)
- Homemade or opened almond milk
- Fresh coconut milk or coconut meat
- Greens: spinach, kale, mixed greens
- Lemons and limes

Freezer

- Banana slices
- Berries, including blackberries, blueberries, raspberries, strawberries
- Frozen greens ($\frac{1}{4}$ to $\frac{1}{2}$ cup or small handful, including spinach, kale, collard greens)

FRUIT-FREE SMOOTHIES

SPA DAY

Chill out, hydrate, and refresh with this spa-day smoothie. It's the perfect way to add a little Zen to your morning.

1 serving vanilla protein powder
$\frac{1}{4}$ to $\frac{1}{2}$ cup diced avocado
1 to 2 tablespoons chia seeds
Juice of $\frac{1}{2}$ to 1 lemon
Fresh mint leaves
Spinach
1 small Persian cucumber
2 cups unsweetened nut milk

Place all the ingredients in a high-speed blender and blend, adding water as needed to reach the desired consistency.

AVOCADO VANILLA LEMON

A squeeze of lemon gives this green smoothie just the right amount of citrusy zest.

1 serving vanilla protein powder
$^1/_4$ avocado
2 tablespoons chia seeds
Squeeze of fresh lemon juice
Handful of spinach
2 cups unsweetened nut milk

Place all the ingredients in a high-speed blender and blend to the desired consistency.

GREEN SMOOTHIE

The original Fab Four Smoothie.

1 serving vanilla protein powder
$^1/_4$ avocado, or 2 tablespoons coconut oil
2 tablespoons chia seeds
Handful of spinach
2 cups unsweetened nut milk

Place all the ingredients in a high-speed blender and blend to the desired consistency.

ALMOND GREEN SMOOTHIE

A filling go-to with a savory sweet finish.

1 serving vanilla protein powder
$^1/_4$ avocado or 2 tablespoons almond butter
2 tablespoons raw fiber
Handful of spinach
2 cups unsweetened nut milk of choice

Place all the ingredients in a high-speed blender and blend to the desired consistency.

MEAN MATCHA

Tastier and healthier than your green tea latte, this smoothie is the perfect mindful boost to get your day started.

1 serving vanilla protein powder
1 to 2 tablespoons MCT oil
1 to 2 tablespoons chia seeds
Spinach
2 to 3 cups unsweetened nut milk
1 serving organic matcha powder

Place all the ingredients in a high-speed blender and blend to the desired consistency.

MOCHA

*Ditch the sugary mocha latte from the coffee shop and enjoy this
smoothie to jump-start your morning or as an afternoon pick-me-up.
The combination of mocha protein powder and coffee makes this rich
smoothie the perfect energy booster, and it keeps you feeling full.*

1 serving mocha protein powder
1 to 2 tablespoons MCT oil
1 to 2 tablespoons chia seeds or flaxseeds
$\frac{1}{4}$ to $\frac{1}{2}$ cup cold brewed coffee (regular or decaf)
2 to 3 cups unsweetened nut milk

Place all the ingredients in a high-speed blender and blend to the desired
consistency.

MINT CHIP

*Unlike most green smoothies, this tastes like a milk shake!
You would never guess something that tastes like a Girl Scout Thin Mint cookie
could be packed with protein and macronutrients.*

1 serving vanilla protein powder
1 to 2 tablespoons MCT oil
1 to 2 tablespoons chia seeds
Fresh mint leaves
2 cups unsweetened nut milk
Cacao nibs, for garnish

Place all the ingredients except the cacao nibs in a high-speed blender and
blend to the desired consistency. Top with cacao nibs.

MOJITO

Mix it up with this riff on a mojito cocktail. It has the tart, minty taste without all the sugar and alcohol, making it a perfect alternative to the real thing.

1 serving vanilla protein powder
1 to 2 tablespoons coconut oil
1 to 2 tablespoons chia seeds
Squeeze of fresh lime juice
Fresh mint leaves
Spinach
2 cups coconut water (unsweetened)

Place all the ingredients in a high-speed blender and blend to the desired consistency.

SNICKERDOODLE

You can finally have cookies for breakfast. Satisfy your holiday sweet tooth with the ultimate guilt-free cinnamon "cookie."

1 serving vanilla protein powder
1 to 2 tablespoons walnut butter
1 to 2 tablespoons flaxseeds
2 to 3 cups unsweetened nut milk
Ground cinnamon and ground nutmeg, for garnish

Place all the ingredients except the cinnamon and nutmeg in a high-speed blender and blend to the desired consistency. Top with cinnamon and nutmeg to taste.

LEMON COOKIE

The combination of sweet and sour in this smoothie creates the perfect healthy lemon cookie.

1 serving vanilla protein powder
1 to 2 tablespoons coconut oil
1 to 2 tablespoons chia seeds, plus more for garnish
Juice of ½ lemon
2 to 3 cups unsweetened nut milk
Lemon zest, for garnish

Place all the ingredients except the lemon zest in a high-speed blender and blend to the desired consistency. Garnish with chia seeds and lemon zest.

LIMEADE

This limeade smoothie is like summertime in a glass. The tart, citrusy flavor of the lime juice balances nicely with the vanilla.

1 serving vanilla protein powder
1 to 2 tablespoons MCT oil or avocado oil
1 to 2 tablespoons chia seeds
Juice of 1 small lime
Spinach
2 to 3 cups unsweetened nut milk
Lime zest, for garnish

Place all the ingredients except the lime zest in a high-speed blender and blend to the desired consistency. Garnish with the lime zest.

GREEN APPLE

Best of Greens brand Green Apple Powder is a blend of organic green superfoods and dark leafy vegetables. The apple taste meshes nicely the coconut flavors in this smoothie.

1 serving vanilla protein powder
1 to 2 tablespoons coconut oil
1 to 2 tablespoons chia seeds
1 tablespoon Best of Greens Green Apple Powder
1 to 2 cups coconut milk

Place all the ingredients in a high-speed blender and blend to the desired consistency.

PEANUT BUTTER CACAO NIB

If you like Reese's peanut butter cups, this is the smoothie for you.

1 serving chocolate protein powder
2 tablespoons peanut butter (or almond butter)
1 to 2 tablespoons chia seeds
2 cups unsweetened nut milk
1 teaspoon cacao nibs

Place all the ingredients in a high-speed blender and blend to the desired consistency.

COCONUT CRÈME

Find your beach and/or your mental hammock with
this creamy, coconutty concoction.

1 serving vanilla protein powder
1 to 2 tablespoons coconut oil
1 to 2 tablespoons chia seeds
1/2 cup coconut meat
2 to 3 cups unsweetened coconut water or unsweetened nut milk
Unsweetened shredded coconut, for garnish

Place all the ingredients except the shredded coconut in a high-speed blender and blend to the desired consistency. Top with shredded coconut.

CHOCOLATE COCONUT

The combination of coconut and chocolate in this smoothie creates a creamy
and rich smoothie that tastes like a milk shake—super decadent!

1 serving chocolate protein powder
1/4 cup unsweetened coconut yogurt
1 to 2 tablespoons chia seeds or flaxseeds
Spinach
2 to 3 cups unsweetened nut milk
Unsweetened shredded coconut, for garnish

Place all the ingredients except the shredded coconut in a high-speed blender and blend to the desired consistency. Garnish with shredded coconut.

DARK CHOCOLATE SEA SALT

Indulge in this decadent chocolate smoothie to start your day.
The sea salt enhances its rich chocolate favor.

1 serving chocolate protein powder
1 to 2 tablespoons MCT oil
1 to 2 tablespoons chia seeds or flaxseeds
2 to 3 cups unsweetened nut milk
Sea salt, for garnish

Place all the ingredients except the sea salt in a high-speed blender and blend
to the desired consistency. Garnish with sea salt.

AVOCADO GREEN DREAM

Avocado in a smoothie? Yes! It offers so much good, healthy fat and helps create a
creamy texture. Get your greens on with this dreamy recipe.

1 serving vanilla protein powder
$\frac{1}{4}$ to $\frac{1}{2}$ avocado
1 to 2 tablespoons chia seeds
Spinach
2 to 3 cups unsweetened coconut water (or green juice)

Place all the ingredients in a high-speed blender and blend to the desired
consistency.

Note: Keep Fab Four Smoothies made with coconut water or green juice, fruit-free. Green juice
should be fruit-free and flavored only with ginger, lemon, or lime.

FRUIT SMOOTHIES

AÇAI GREEN

Antioxidants abound in this balanced smoothie that won't skyrocket your blood sugar the way açai bowls will!

1 serving vanilla protein powder
1 to 2 tablespoons organic almond butter
1 to 2 tablespoons chia or flaxseeds
Organic açai (a freeze-dried serving of 20 calories)
2 cups unsweetened almond milk
Handful of spinach

Place all the ingredients in a high-speed blender and blend to the desired consistency.

BLUEBERRY MUFFIN

Skip that sugar-loaded muffin and try this sweet smoothie instead. The nut butter and blueberries pair nicely to re-create the comforting flavor of a blueberry muffin.

1 serving vanilla protein powder
1 to 2 tablespoons nut butter of choice
1 serving raw fiber powder
$\frac{1}{4}$ cup frozen or fresh blueberries, plus more for garnish
2 to 3 cups unsweetened nut milk
Hemp seeds, for garnish

Place all the ingredients except the hemp seeds in a high-speed blender and blend to the desired consistency. If you use fresh blueberries, add a few ice cubes before blending to cool. Garnish with hemp seeds and blueberries.

151

BLUEBERRY COCONUT CRÈME

A sweet and creamy blend of two of my favorite foods, this smoothie is a great way to balance yourself at breakfast or in the afternoon.

1 serving vanilla protein powder
1/4 cup frozen or fresh blueberries
2 tablespoons unsweetened shredded coconut
2 tablespoons coconut oil
2 cups unsweetened vanilla almond milk

Place all the ingredients in a high-speed blender and blend to the desired consistency. If you use fresh blueberries, add a few ice cubes before blending to cool.

BERRY GREEN

Adding berries to your green smoothie is the perfect way to include a little sweetness in a refreshing breakfast.

1 serving vanilla protein powder
1 to 2 tablespoons MCT oil
1 to 2 tablespoons chia seeds or flaxseeds
1/4 cup frozen or fresh mixed berries
Spinach
Kale
Parsley

Place all the ingredients in a high-speed blender and blend, adding 2 to 3 cups water to reach the desired consistency. If you use fresh berries, add a few ice cubes before blending to cool.

ALMOND BUTTER AND RASPBERRY JAM

Jam out with this scrumptious and hearty combination of nutty and berry flavors.

1 serving vanilla protein powder

1 to 2 tablespoons organic almond butter

1 to 2 tablespoons chia seeds or flaxseeds

$\frac{1}{4}$ cup fresh or frozen raspberries

2 cups unsweetened almond milk

> Place all the ingredients in a high-speed blender and blend to the desired consistency. If you use fresh raspberries, add a few ice cubes before blending to cool.

PEANUT BUTTER AND JELLY

What could be better than PB&J in a cup? This smoothie is reminiscent of that classic childhood sandwich, but will also keep you satiated for hours.

1 serving vanilla protein powder

1 to 2 tablespoons organic peanut butter

1 to 2 tablespoons chia seeds or flaxseeds

$\frac{1}{4}$ cup fresh or frozen strawberries

2 cups unsweetened nut milk

> Place all the ingredients in a high-speed blender and blend to the desired consistency. If you use fresh strawberries, add a few ice cubes before blending to cool.

STRAWBERRY SHORTCAKE

Full of sweet and creamy flavor, this smoothie is a healthy and
tasty alternative to strawberry shortcake.

1 serving vanilla protein powder
Coconut cream
1 to 2 tablespoons chia seeds, plus more for garnish
¼ cup diced frozen or fresh strawberries
2 to 3 cups unsweetened nut milk

Place all the ingredients in a high-speed blender and blend to the desired consistency. If you use fresh strawberries, add a few ice cubes before blending to cool. Garnish with chia seeds.

STRAWBERRY BASIL

This pleasant, aromatic smoothie is like a summer salad in a glass.

1 serving vanilla protein powder
1 tablespoon MCT oil
2 tablespoons chia seeds
¼ cup diced frozen or fresh strawberries
Handful of spinach
Handful of basil
2 cups unsweetened almond milk

Place all the ingredients in a high-speed blender and blend to the desired consistency. If you use fresh strawberries, add a few ice cubes before blending to cool.

STRAWBERRY GREEN

Get your greens while you satisfy your taste buds with this simple recipe.

1 serving vanilla protein powder
2 tablespoons MCT oil
1 to 2 tablespoons chia seeds
$\frac{1}{4}$ cup frozen or fresh strawberries
2 to 3 cups unsweetened nut milk
Handful of spinach

Place all the ingredients in a high-speed blender and blend to the desired consistency.

CHOCOLATE-DIPPED STRAWBERRY

An indulgent play on that special Valentine's Day dessert.

1 serving chocolate protein powder
1 to 2 tablespoons fat of choice
1 to 2 tablespoons chia seeds or flaxseeds
$\frac{1}{4}$ cup diced frozen or fresh strawberries
2 to 3 cups unsweetened nut milk

Place all the ingredients in a high-speed blender and blend to the desired consistency. If you use fresh strawberries, add a few ice cubes before blending to cool.

APPLES AND ALMOND BUTTER

If you enjoy snacking on apple slices and almond butter, this is the smoothie is for you! And it has a hint of apple pie.

1 serving vanilla protein powder
1 to 2 tablespoons almond butter
1 to 2 tablespoons chia seeds or flaxseeds
1 cored apple
Spinach
2 to 3 cups unsweetened nut milk
Ground cinnamon, ground nutmeg, and walnuts, for garnish

Place all the ingredients except the cinnamon, nutmeg, and walnuts in a high-speed blender and blend to the desired consistency. Garnish with cinnamon, nutmeg, and walnuts.

CARAMEL APPLE PIE

This treat of a smoothie will satisfy the county-fairgoer in you, all the while setting you up for four to six hours of blood sugar balance.

1 serving vanilla protein powder
2 tablespoons MCT oil or almond butter
1 tablespoon flaxseeds
$\frac{1}{2}$ large or 1 small date
$\frac{1}{4}$ green apple, cored
2 cups unsweetened nut milk

Place all the ingredients in a high-speed blender and blend to the desired consistency.

LEAN AND GREEN

A no-frills green metabolism booster, with a sweet little apple kick.

1 serving vanilla protein powder
1 to 2 tablespoons chia seeds
2 tablespoons avocado oil
2 cups chopped kale
$\frac{1}{4}$ green apple, cored
1 cup unsweetened almond milk
2 to 4 ice cubes

> Place all the ingredients in a high-speed blender and blend to the desired consistency.

CUCUMBER KALE APPLE AVOCADO

Get your system moving with this well-balanced green machine.

1 serving vanilla protein powder
1 tablespoon MCT oil
$\frac{1}{2}$ avocado
$\frac{1}{2}$ cup cucumber
$\frac{1}{4}$ apple
Handful of kale

> Place all the ingredients and 2 cups water in a high-speed blender and blend to the desired consistency.

APPLE PIE

*With only a handful of ingredients and a couple of seconds in the blender, you can
re-create a healthy version of a comforting apple pie. Pair it with a summer day on the
porch or a cozy winter day in front of the fire.*

1 serving vanilla protein powder
1 to 2 tablespoons organic almond butter
1 to 2 tablespoons flaxseeds
$^1/_2$ apple
2 cups unsweetened nut milk
Dash of ground cinnamon
Dash of ground nutmeg

Place all the ingredients in a high-speed blender and blend to the desired
consistency.

WATERMELON MINT

*This refreshing play on a watermelon agua fresca, with a hint of mint,
is one of my summer go-tos.*

1 serving vanilla protein powder
1 to 2 tablespoons MCT oil
1 to 2 tablespoons chia seeds, plus more for garnish
$^1/_4$ cup cubed watermelon
Fresh mint leaves, plus more for garnish
2 cups unsweetened nut milk

Place all the ingredients in a high-speed blender and blend to the desired
consistency. Garnish with mint leaves and chia seeds.

CHUNKY MONKEY

This recipe checks a lot of boxes with a delicious combination of peanut butter, banana, and chocolate. Try it the next time you're craving a sweet breakfast or an indulgent dessert.

1 serving chocolate protein powder
1 to 2 tablespoons peanut or almond butter
1 tablespoon chia seeds or flaxseeds
½ banana
Handful of spinach
2 to 3 cups unsweetened nut milk
Slivered almonds, for garnish

Place all the ingredients except the almonds in a high-speed blender and blend to the desired consistency. Garnish with the almonds.

BANANA BREAD

For anyone who loves a slice of warm banana bread but is searching for a healthy alternative, this is it. The nuttiness of this smoothie perfectly complements the banana, making it great for breakfast or even a healthy dessert.

1 serving vanilla protein powder
1 to 2 tablespoons walnut butter
1 to 2 tablespoons flaxseeds
½ banana
2 to 3 cups unsweetened nut milk
Ground cinnamon, ground nutmeg, and chopped walnuts, for garnish

Place all the ingredients except the cinnamon, nutmeg, and walnuts in a high-speed blender and blend to the desired consistency. Garnish with the cinnamon, nutmeg, and walnuts.

SALTED CARAMEL

Salted caramel in a healthy way? Yes, please! This smoothie is decadent like a milk shake but still full of protein, fiber, and fat to keep you satiated.

1 serving vanilla protein powder
1 to 2 tablespoons MCT oil
1 serving raw fiber powder
1 small date
2 cups unsweetened nut milk
$1/2$ teaspoon pink Himalayan salt or coarse sea salt, for garnish

Place all the ingredients except the salt in a high-speed blender and blend to the desired consistency. Garnish with the salt.

OATMEAL RAISIN

Taking the nutritious elements of an oatmeal cookie and blending them together creates a delicious, fiber-rich, and protein-packed smoothie.

1 serving vanilla protein powder
1 to 2 tablespoons nut butter of choice
1 serving raw fiber powder
2 tablespoons raisins
2 to 3 cups unsweetened nut milk
Ground cinnamon and ground nutmeg, for garnish

Place all the ingredients except the cinnamon and nutmeg in a high-speed blender and blend to the desired consistency. Garnish with the cinnamon and nutmeg.

MANGO KALE MADNESS

Channel some island vibes and change up your ordinary green smoothie with the tropical flavor of mango.

1 serving vanilla protein powder
1 to 2 tablespoons MCT oil or avocado oil
1 tablespoon chia seeds
$\frac{1}{4}$ cup frozen or fresh mango
Kale
2 to 3 cups unsweetened coconut water

Place all the ingredients in a high-speed blender and blend to the desired consistency. If you use fresh mango, add a few ice cubes before blending to cool.

CHOCOLATE CHERRY

A healthy spin on a milk shake, this smoothie is packed with protein and the rich flavors of chocolate and cherry.

1 serving chocolate protein powder
1 to 2 tablespoons MCT oil
1 to 2 tablespoons chia seeds or flaxseeds, plus more for garnish
$\frac{1}{4}$ cup frozen or fresh pitted cherries
2 to 3 cups unsweetened nut milk
Lemon zest and chia seeds, for garnish

Place all the ingredients except the lemon zest and chia seeds in a high-speed blender and blend to the desired consistency. If you use fresh cherries, add a few ice cubes before blending to cool. Garnish with the lemon zest and chia seeds.

CHERRY CACAO

When in season, fresh cherries are one of my favorite farmers' market buys. Their sweetness helps make this smoothie pop.

1 serving vanilla protein powder
1 tablespoon almond butter
1 tablespoon MCT oil
1 tablespoon chia seeds
1/4 cup frozen or fresh pitted cherries
Handful of spinach
1 cup unsweetened nut milk
Cacao nibs, for garnish

Place all the ingredients except the cacao nibs in a high-speed blender and blend to the desired consistency. Garnish with cacao nibs.

PANCAKE PARTY

Tap into your inner child with this ode to Saturdays past.

1 serving vanilla protein powder
1 to 2 tablespoons nut butter of choice
1 serving raw fiber powder
1/3 banana (optional)
2 to 3 cups unsweetened nut milk
1 teaspoon Lakanto Maple Flavored Sugar-Free Syrup

Place all the ingredients except the maple syrup in a high-speed blender and blend to the desired consistency. Garnish with the maple syrup.

PEACHES AND GREENS

The peach in this smoothie makes a sweet, creamy base that perfectly complements the coconut and greens.

1 serving vanilla protein powder
1 to 2 tablespoons coconut oil
1 to 2 tablespoons chia seeds or flaxseeds
$\frac{1}{4}$ cup frozen or fresh sliced peaches, plus cubed peaches for garnish
Spinach
2 to 3 cups unsweetened nut milk
Coconut cream, for garnish (optional)

Place all the ingredients except the coconut cream (if using) in a high-speed blender and blend to the desired consistency. If you use fresh peaches, add a few ice cubes before blending to cool. Garnish with the cubed peaches and coconut cream.

PUMPKIN PIE

Start Thanksgiving Day with this festive smoothie and lose the urge to gorge at feast time. Perfect for any fall day, too!

1 serving vanilla protein powder
1 tablespoon flaxseeds
1 tablespoon MCT oil
2 cups unsweetened almond milk
1 teaspoon ground cinnamon
1 teaspoon ground nutmeg
$\frac{1}{2}$ cup pure pumpkin puree

Place all the ingredients in a high-speed blender and blend to the desired consistency.

FUNCTIONAL SUPERFOOD SMOOTHIES

ASHWAGANDHA GREEN SMOOTHIE

Combat stress and cortisol with the help of ashwagandha, a powerful medicinal herb that can also help with fatigue, lack of energy, and mental acuity.

1 serving vanilla protein powder
1 to 2 tablespoons coconut oil or MCT oil
1 to 2 tablespoons chia seeds
$^1/_2$ to 1 teaspoon ashwagandha
Handful of spinach
2 cups unsweetened almond milk
$^1/_4$ cup frozen or fresh blueberries

Place all the ingredients in a high-speed blender and blend to the desired consistency, adding a few ice cubes before blending if desired.

KALE AND HEMP HEARTS

Hemp hearts (raw shelled hemp seeds) are a superfood with protein, essential fatty acids, and micronutrients such as iron and vitamin E.

1 serving vanilla protein powder
1 tablespoon almond butter
2 tablespoons chia seeds

Handful of kale
1 tablespoon MCT oil
1 teaspoon ashwagandha
2 cups unsweetened almond milk
Hemp hearts, for garnish

Place all the ingredients except the hemp hearts in a high-speed blender and blend to the desired consistency. Garnish with the hemp hearts.

GREEN RHOAD TO HEALTH

This green smoothie is another de-stress powerhouse that also assists with weight loss and boosts overall nutrition.

1 serving vanilla protein powder
1 to 2 tablespoons almond butter
1 to 2 tablespoons chia seeds
$1/2$ to 1 teaspoon Rhodiola
Handful of spinach
$1/4$ cup microgreens
2 cups unsweetened almond milk

Place all the ingredients in a high-speed blender and blend to the desired consistency.

CHAGA CACAO

Chaga is a nutrient-dense mushroom that's full of antioxidants. Ground yourself and help your immune system with this healthy smoothie. Get a little cacao to boot!

1 serving vanilla protein powder
1 to 2 tablespoons almond butter
1 to 2 tablespoons chia seeds
$\frac{1}{2}$ to 1 teaspoon chaga
2 cups unsweetened almond milk
Cacao nibs, for garnish

Place all the ingredients except the cacao nibs in a high-speed blender and blend to the desired consistency. Garnish with the cacao nibs.

TURMERIC PUMPKIN SPICE

This delectable smoothie fights inflammation and gives your brain and body an overall chill because of serotonin-boosting properties in the tryptophan found in pumpkin seeds!

$1\frac{1}{2}$ cups unsweetened almond milk
1 serving vanilla protein powder
1 tablespoon MCT oil
1 tablespoon chia seeds
$1\frac{1}{2}$ teaspoons Ceylon cinnamon
$\frac{1}{2}$ teaspoon ground cloves

1 teaspoon Gaia Golden Milk (or 1 teaspoon turmeric and a pinch of black pepper)

$^1/_2$ cup frozen pumpkin puree

1 to 3 drops Pumpkin Spice stevia (optional)

1 tablespoon pumpkin seeds, to garnish

Place all the ingredients except the pumpkin seeds in a high-speed blender and blend to the desired consistency. Garnish with pumpkin seeds if desired.

MACUNA CHAI SMOOTHIE

You're going to love macuna—this dopamine-boosting amino acid will help regulate your moods while the cinnamon will help balance your blood sugar by increasing your insulin sensitivity.

1 cup unsweetened almond milk

1 serving vanilla protein

1 tablespoon chia seeds

1 tablespoon cashew butter

1 teaspoon vanilla extract

$^1/_2$ teaspoon ground Ceylon cinnamon

$^1/_4$ teaspoon ground ginger

$^1/_8$ teaspoon ground nutmeg

$^1/_8$ teaspoon ground cardamom

Pinch of ground cloves

Place all the ingredients in a high-speed blender and blend to the desired consistency.

FAB FOUR WINTER BERRY

Body + Eden takes Chinese herbs to the next level, fermenting them with probiotics and adding in the ashwagandha, which boosts your immune system and offers you another powerful de-stressing agent.

1 cup unsweetened vanilla almond milk
1 tablespoon Four Sigmatic Smoothie Shroomer
$\frac{1}{8}$ tsp. Body + Eden Immunity Herbal Tonic
1 serving vanilla pea protein
$\frac{1}{4}$ cup frozen cranberries
Handful of spinach
1 tablespoon coconut oil
1 tablespoon chia seeds

Place all the ingredients in a high-speed blender and blend to the desired consistency.

BANANA NUT BREAD SMOOTHIE

A little bit sweet, this super smoothie will support gut repair and the ongoing health of your GI system.

1 cup unsweetened vanilla almond milk
1 serving of collagen
1 tablespoon walnut butter
1 teaspoon acacia fiber
$\frac{1}{2}$ banana

Place all the ingredients in a high-speed blender and blend to the desired consistency.

GINGERSNAP SMOOTHIE

Ranking higher on the ORAC scale than açai and turmeric, clove packs a powerful antioxidant punch. This smoothie will help you fight oxidative stress, protect against free radicals, and give your system a natural cleanse of toxic buildup.

1 1/2 cups unsweetened almond milk
1 serving vanilla protein
1/2 banana, peeled, sliced, and frozen
1/4 teaspoon ground ginger
1/4 teaspoon clove
1 to 3 drops English Toffee stevia
1 cap of Liquid Light or 1 teaspoon food-grade diatomaceous earth (silica)

Place all the ingredients in a high-speed blender and blend to the desired consistency.

A WEEK OF BODY LOVE

Although no week in my life is quite the same, I do tend to follow certain routines and rituals to make sure I feel my best. This *Body Love* Week captures me from Monday through Sunday and shows how easy it can be to eat well without a fuss, while at the same time enjoying life, getting in some fun, sweaty workouts, and relaxing.

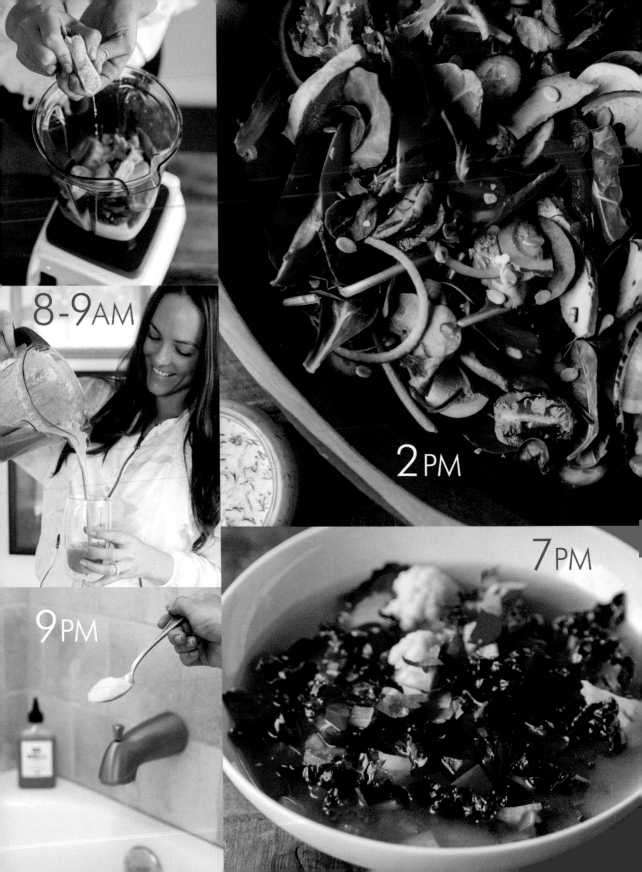

8-9AM

2PM

7PM

9PM

MONDAY

Start the Week Sweaty!

7 AM: Super Sweaty Workout Class (Spin or HIIT)

I might not work out every day, but I love to start the week with a class (either Sunday night or Monday morning). In fact, I prefer to do my hard workouts (Spin or HIIT) on Mondays and Fridays to bookend my week, which also helps me make sure every week has at least two sweaty workouts!

8-9 AM Breakfast: Upgraded Spa Smoothie

See page 142 for a refreshing, nutrient-dense smoothie that will start your week off right. Lemon and cucumbers contain hydrating, nourishing and astringent properties that are very good for skin on the inside and outside. My spa smoothie incorporates both beauty foods plus avocado for added healthy fat. Any Fab Four smoothie can be upgraded for more nutrition by adding sugar-free superfood powders that are antioxidant, vitamin, and mineral rich, such as turmeric, green powders, mushrooms, or adaptogens (page 139).

2 PM Lunch: Chicken Chop Salad with Herby Ranch

A big chicken salad is a quick lunch when you use an easy Sunday prep rotisserie and farmer's market chopped veggies. To accompany, spike a big glass of water with a squeeze of lemon, splash

of apple cider vinegar or one of my favorite nutrient packets: Oxylent, 8G, or NUUN.

7 PM Dinner: Bone Broth Vegetable Soup

Looking to autocorrect from a weekend of fun? No need to be drastic. Instead, love your body with nourishing food! Bone broth (see page 107) is easy to digest and loaded with rich minerals that support the immune system, heal the gut, and reduce inflammation.

9 PM: Epsom Salt Bath or Scrub

Occasionally, I need to relax in an Epsom salt bath (1 cup Epsom salt and a few drops of essential oils) to nip Monday's stress in the bud. Just 15 to 20 minutes in a warm bath calms the nervous system and reminds me to take a few deep cleansing breaths to prepare my body for bed.

Honestly, it's all about carving just a little me time out and listening close enough to hear what I need in the moments of down time. This kind of routine helps me get the sleep I need to restore body and brain!

10 PM at latest: Early Bed Time

It's tempting to stay up late to get control of your inbox but just like your morning workout, starting the week with eight solid hours of sleep can help you get your body on an even keel for the rest of the week.

TUESDAY

7 AM

From meeting clients to building healthy content, being camera ready is part of the job! Lately I've become obsessed with the Honest Beauty brand. I was never able to wear foundation without looking greasy, dealing with breakouts, or just feeling bad about swiping chemicals on my face. With Honest Everything tinted moisturizer and cream blush and a swipe of gluten-free mascara (I keep trying different brands!)—I am good to go!

Tip: Gluten in mascara is volumizing but for years it caused me to get little red circles at the corners of my eyes. Now they are gone!

8 AM Breakfast:
Decadent Fab Four Smoothie

Craving a bit of sugar? Start your day with a decadent cacao rich Fab Four smoothie to satisfy those cravings before they hit. Raw cacao is packed full of flavonoids and contains four times the antioxidants of traditional cocoa powder. This "super-antioxidant" even ranks higher on the ORAC score than acai berries, spinach, blueberries and even green tea. Try Vanilla Chocolate Chip (pictured, use Mint Chip recipe on page 145 without the mint) or Dark Chocolate Sea Salt (page 150).

12:30 PM Lunch:
Fab Four Variety

All my meals and smoothies are made up of four crucial ingredients—fat, fiber, protein, and greens. I call this combination my Fab Four! But you might be amazed at how you can get the Fab Four into easy-to-make lunches. Try veggies and dips, spicy nori burritos, or wrap up your favorite salad in a dehydrated zucchini wrap. This delicious French Salmon Salad with Cucumber Chips and Smashed Avocado is one of my faves!

4 PM Afternoon Pick Me Up:
Turmeric Latte

Turmeric not only contains antioxidant, anti-inflammatory, antiviral, antibacterial, antifungal, and anticancer properties—it can also benefit your waistline, balancing blood sugar by slowing down the metabolism of carbohydrates after meals.

6 PM Workout: Yoga

I love yoga more than any other workout; it's a moving meditation that makes my whole being feel calm and elated at the same time. It tones and lengthens the muscles while aligning the skeleton.

8 PM Dinner: Taco Tuesday!
Lettuce-Wrapped Tacos
(with protein of choice)

Having grown up on the beach in Southern California, I'll add guacamole to almost anything, including salads, bowls, or lettuce- or jicama-wrapped tacos (see page 118)! Mix in your protein of choice (such as chicken, grass-finished beef, fish, or shrimp) and top with your favorite fat sauce (page 125).

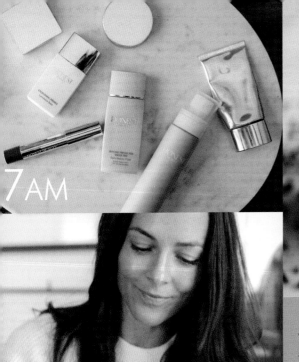

7AM

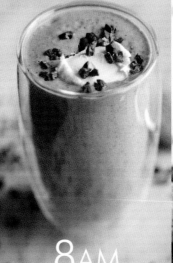

8AM

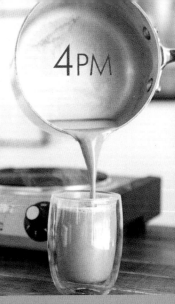

4PM

12:30PM

HERBILICIOUS!

You don't need to eat a salad to get the medicinal benefits of greens! Simply add herbs. Check out these amazing benefits of herbs—and note that microgreens (no more than 14 days post-germination are up to 40 times higher in nutrients!

CILANTRO: Chelates heavy metal from the body
BASIL: Anti-inflammatory, anticancer, and antibacterial
PARSLEY: Neutralizes carcinogens
ROSEMARY: Improves circulation and digestion
DILL: Antidepressive, increases energy, and protects
        against free radicals

8PM

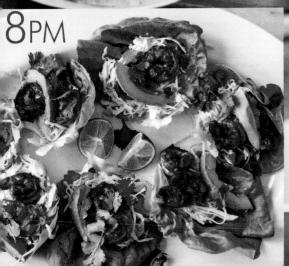

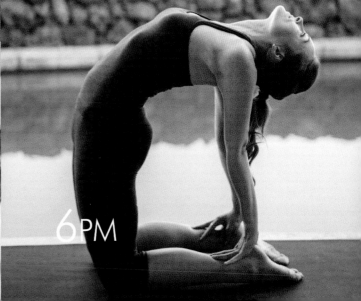

6PM

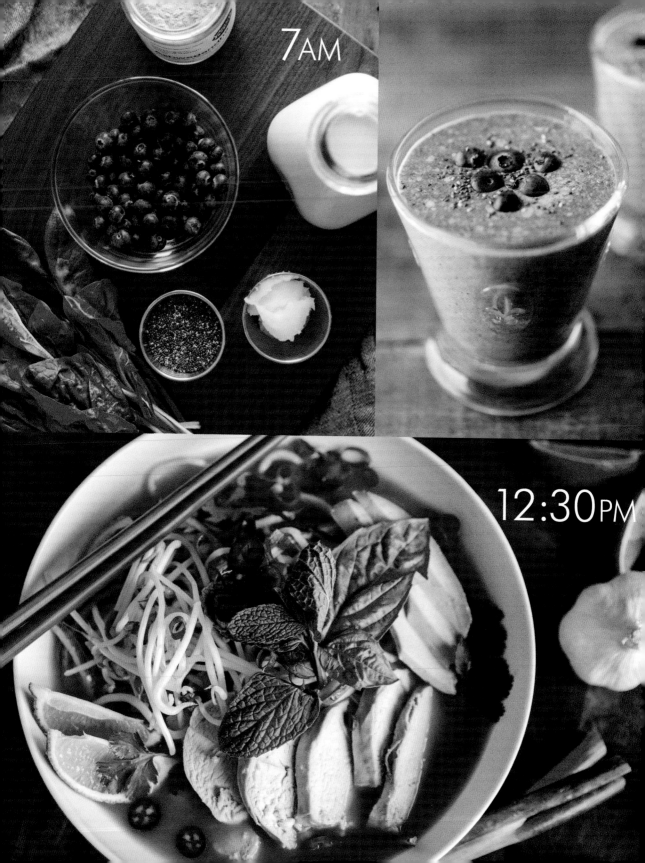

7AM

12:30PM

WEDNESDAY

Turn Around Hump Day with Some Fun!

7 AM Breakfast:
Blueberry Muffin Smoothie
with Coconut Oil and
Ashwagandha
(page 151)

Don't let not having fresh produce deter you from making your smoothie—frozen wild blueberries and organic spinach are more affordable, preserve vitamins, and also cool down your smoothie! Ashwagandha (powder or liquid) comes from a potent root and can calm the body and its nervous system.

MAGNESIUM TO THE RESCUE!

MAGNESIUM: Any chance you suffer from constipation? Are the symptoms worse when you eat out with friends or travel? Keep things moving by taking a daily recommended amount of oxidized magnesium before bed after you've been eating a little less clean!

12:30 PM

It doesn't need to be cold outside to enjoy some hearty, delicious soup or chili—try a Fake Pho or Bison Chili for a delicious dose of nutrition. Bison is the perfect iron and folate source for a healthy pregnancy; delivers antioxidant omega 3 fatty acids and vitamin E for a glow from the inside out, and is loaded with zinc and selenium, two must-have minerals for thyroid health.

7 PM Dinner:
Girls' Night Dinner

Time with friends is absolutely part of the Body Love program! I advise my clients to get out and connect with their friends, laugh, love, and be social. Community plays a huge role in lowering stress, increasing longevity, and making us happy! Suggest a clean location and pair a protein with a few vegetable sides. No need to be "good" by restricting yourself to a salad! My go-to dinner out is fish and veggies plus one glass of Pinot Noir.

THURSDAY

7 AM Morning Wake Up: Cucumber Lemon Water

Waking up your body and brain means rehydration. Cucumbers reduce puffiness under eyes and internally. The cucumber will release quercetin, a flavonoid antioxidant that helps reduce swelling.

8 AM: Morning Walk

Morning movement is meditative for me. It allows me to purge stress, plan my daily inbox attack, and see the forest from the trees. Depending on the weather, I might take a nice walk, do a yoga flow, or head to the gym for a simple workout class.

9 AM Breakfast: Macuna Chai Smoothie (page 167)

This smoothie combines mellow vanilla flavor with fragrant cinnamon and deep, rich notes of clove—a spice that doesn't get enough love! Cloves deliver antioxidants to fight free radicals, give you more than 100 percent of your daily value of vitamin C, vitamin K, and manganese, and possess anti-inflammatory and pain-killing properties.

12:30 PM: Lunch: Pesto Zoodles and Marinara Turkey Meatballs

Poor night's sleep? Craving carbs? Load your favorite squash zoodles with a fat sauce such as pesto, cashew alfredo, or a sugar free marinara.

And make sure you hydrate with ACV Water—just add a tablespoon of apple cider vinegar (ACV) to a glass of water. ACV is a liver and lymphatic tonic that can help detox your body.

5 PM: Afternoon Freeze or Sweat

Cryotherapy is localized or whole-body exposure to subzero temperatures to decrease inflammation, increase cellular survival, decrease pain and spasms, and promote overall health.

Another detox I enjoy is a quiet sit in an *infrared sauna* as afternoon flows into evening. One of my favorite treats, a sauna can help burn calories, make you sweat, speed up your metabolism, relieve muscle pain, improve the immune system, remove toxins, help the appearance of cellulite, and ease joint pain and stiffness.

7 PM Dinner: Fish Pocket

Aim to have fish a couple times a week. Wild salmon is one of the best food sources for omega-3 fatty acids and protein. Omega 3 deficiencies contribute to chronic acne, and adequate levels of this anti-inflammatory fatty acid will not only keep your skin clear but also increase cell hydration from the inside out. Wild salmon is also known for being rich in vitamin D and selenium, which protect the skin from the sun's harmful UV rays. Sardines, oysters, and mackerel also supply Omega 3s, an awesome beauty builder.

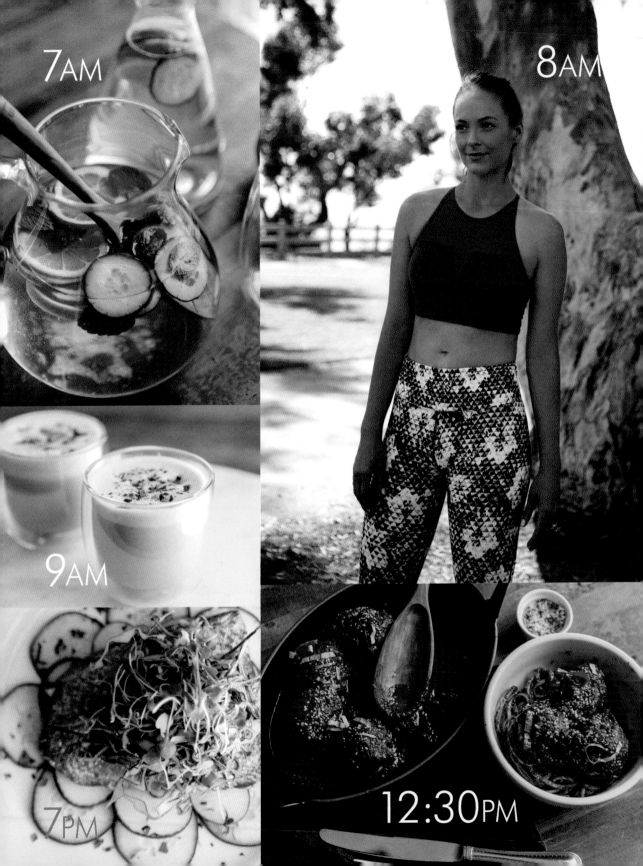

7AM

8AM

9AM

7PM

12:30PM

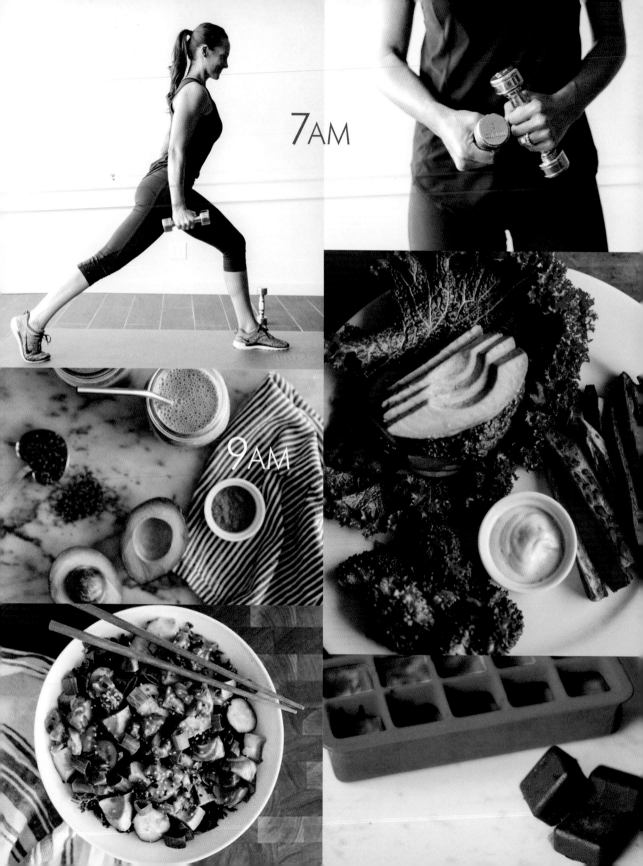

7AM

9AM

FRIDAY

7 AM:
HIIT Workout

The weekend can be a wild card, so just as on Monday, I try to do a hard workout on Friday. Starting and closing the week by getting nice and sweaty will energize and calm you! A tough HIIT workout also fires up your metabolism ahead of time, in case you'd like to indulge in a couple of weekend splurges.

9 AM Breakfast:
Coco Creamy
Matcha Smoothie

Matcha tea contains catechin EGCg (epigallocatechin gallate) a potent cancer-fighting antioxidant that counteracts the damaging effects of free radicals caused by pollution, UV rays, radiation, and chemicals, which can lead to cell and DNA damage. Further, the L-Theanine in green tea is known to increase focus and concentration. Always look for 100 percent Organic Matcha powder to avoid lead toxicity.

1 PM Lunch:
Out with Coworkers or Friends

Find yourself ordering bad takeout at lunch? Make your own healthy menu of all the local takeout locations and your favorite clean orders. Instead of pulling up the entire menu online and caving to something you don't really want to eat, grab your personal menu PDF and choose from your healthy picks!

7:30 PM Dinner:
Burger Night!

I love celebrating Friday with a burger bar, complete with baked sweet potato and parsnip fries. Sometimes I enjoy my burger wrapped in lettuce or use roasted sweet potatoes (sliced in circles) as a bun!

POST-DINNER TREAT
Freezer Fudge Bite
(page 134)

This delicious treat is so satisfying. Make a whole batch and enjoy for days!

SATURDAY

10 AM: Brunch

I love to wake up slowly on a Saturday and enjoy a homemade breaky! I keep my Fab Four in mind, of course, but give myself some extra room to enjoy and have some fun. Some of my favorite breakfasts are Warm Chia Pudding, Protein Pancakes, Coconut Yogurt Bowl, Avocado Japanese Yam "Toast," or a *big* smoothie bowl with extra toppings!

1 PM: Mid-Day Play

I love to hit the beach for a refreshing surf, hike a hill, or find a set of local stairs. This kind of playful exercise is an easy way to get in your exercise. You can even clock 10,000 steps while jamming around your local outdoor mall in search of sales or get in your garden for some manual labor. Be in contact with the earth, let the sun hit your face, and play.

4 PM Pre-Night Out Plan

Looking for something to hold you over until your night out? Have a Roadie (page 200) or half a Fab Four smoothie or opt for a detox salad full of greens. Just as you'd avoid the grocery store when you're starving, it's important to never go to a big social gathering like a cocktail party, wedding, or sports event hungry. Take a plain shake "roadie" in the car with you and arrive with balanced blood sugar and a solid liquid base. Try any one of my basic shakes to help you avoid eating fried appetizers, getting tipsy off your first cocktail or eating something that doesn't make you feel great.

8 PM Night Out:
Wedding, Shower, Double Date, Football Game, Concert, or Sushi!

You can't plan your meals every night, so when I know I'm going out on the town, I simply keep in some easy swaps in mind (see page 197 for some great ones).

If you're having Asian food, including sushi, swap gluten-free, soy-free, MSG-free coconut aminos for soy sauce or tamari. This salty replacement contains 17 amino acids and B vitamins and also saves you 700 mg of sodium, dropping your intake from 36 percent to a mere 5 percent—bloaty sushi hangover be gone!

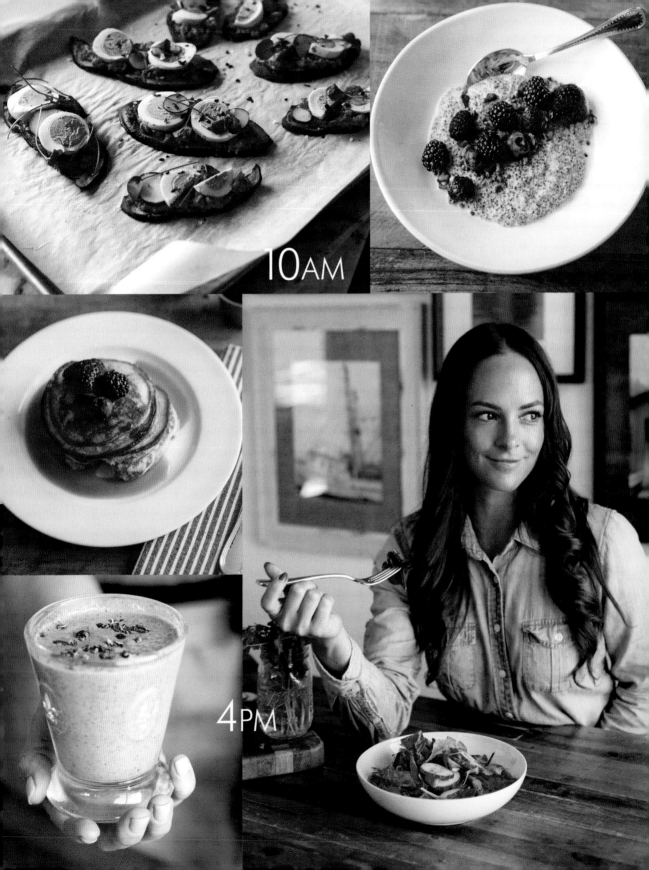

10AM

4PM

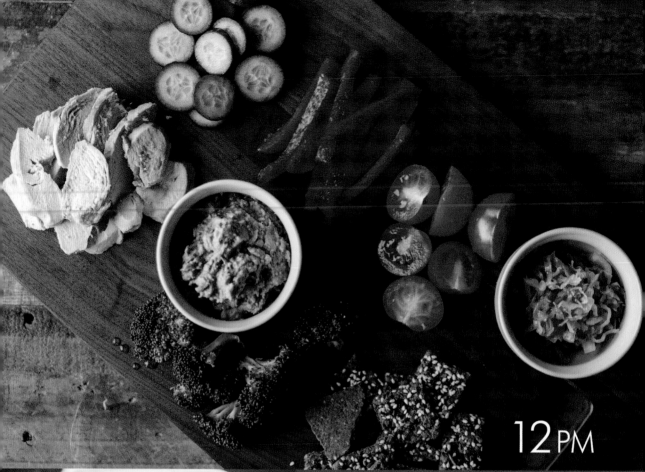

12 PM

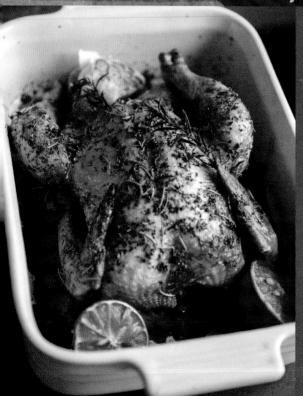

SUNDAY SELF CARE:
What do you need?

Sunday has long been considered a day of rest. Take this tradition to heart by tuning in and making sure you're taking care of yourself—mind, body, and soul. I trust that I will be in a rested, calm place, ready for the week ahead if I've included some of these during the week:

- Exercise: 2 or 3 days a week
- Yoga: at least twice a week
- Meditation
- Cryotherapy or sauna
- Massage

SUNDAY

Choose Your Own Adventure!

Hit the farmer's market and buy a fresh piece of fruit for a seasonal smoothie flavor. If you go before brunch, have a smoothie first. If you go after, wake up slowly, have a fatty coffee or tea, and head to brunch.

10 AM: Brunch

Although most weekdays I recommend that my clients start with a fiber- and protein-rich smoothie, when the weekend hits, go ahead and enjoy the warm satisfaction of a brunch without deprivation. Of course our overall goals remain the same: stabilize blood sugar with protein and fat. What contains both? Eggs! I love poached eggs over an arugula salad or a big veggie omelet with almond milk cheese (Kite Hill is a great brand!). Not only are the whites full of protein but egg yolks are one of the richest dietary sources of the B-complex vitamin choline, which promotes better neurological function, reduced inflammation, and improved mood.

12 PM: Light Prep for the Week (Optional)

Not everyone likes to prep for the week ahead, so this tip isn't mandatory but it can help save you time throughout the week. On Sundays, I love to prep some staple meal-builders that can be turned into easy go-to meals:

- Roast or buy one rotisserie chicken
- Prep French Salmon Salad (page 121)
- Hard-boil 3 to 6 eggs
- Chop all sorts of veggies to add to salads or to-go snacks
- Make a Thai Peanut salad (lasts in the fridge; page 124)
- Prep or purchase (frozen) bone broth (page 107)

2 PM: Yoga Workout

I love to close my week with a yoga flow, either at a nearby class or on my own at home.

OPTION 1
4 PM

Late Lunch or Early Dinner: Sunday Health Plate Flexibility is the key to success! I grew up on "health plates" and when I was little that meant a plate of crackers, cheese, turkey, and apples. Today, I still enjoy my childhood favorites, but now it's in an elevated way—my simple Fab Four health plate includes my favorite fat dips, proteins, fibrous vegetables, and greens! It's the perfect late lunch for a Sunday football game when you feel like snacking and a great way to get loads of colors on your plate. Load your plate with sliced avocado, flax crackers, hummus, blanched broccoli florets, microgreens, cucumber florets, almond butter, celery sticks, fermented vegetables (such sauerkraut or kimchi), and sliced cooked chicken, turkey, or steak.

OPTION 2

Special Sunday Dinner

On some Sundays, I love spending a little more time and preparing a special dinner. It's the night I recipe test, get creative, make comfort food, or knock off one of my takeout favorites, such as Pho, Broccoli Beef, or Shepherd's Pie.

Plan to be done eating by 6 pm on Sunday night, then go for a fruit-free smoothie (see the Spa Smoothie on Monday!) Monday morning to let your body cleanse itself of excess insulin and autocorrect from the fun! Instead of focusing on food, refocus on self-care.

8 PM: Sunday Night Slow Down

Ending the week is all about slowing down, dimming the lights, calming my mind, and taking a hot second to listen to what I need. To set the mood, I illuminate my Himalayan Crystal Rock Salt Lamp, slip into cozies, and brew a cup of tea. When my stress level is especially high, I lean on adaptogenic teas from Four Sigma Foods, Moon Juice, or Sun Potion or a magnesium drink such as Natural Calm to help me relax and sleep more deeply.

Loving your body does not take extra time! You can cruise through your week when you get into a flow of prepping your Fab Four and smoothies, making sure you sneak in some exercise, and always giving yourself some R&R!

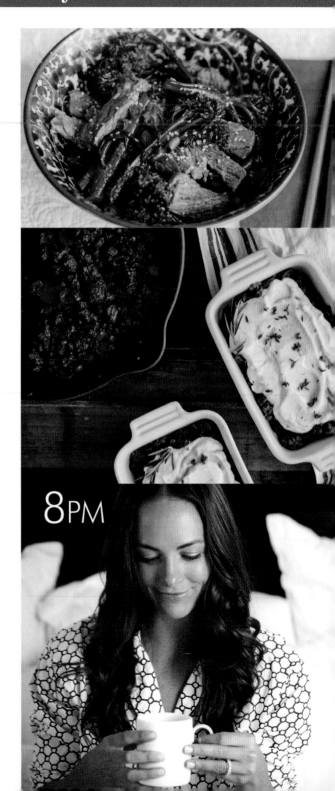

8PM

PART
THREE

YOUR
FAB FOUR
LIFE

8

LIVING THE FAB FOUR LIFE

"THIS IS SO EASY!" That's one of the most common texts I receive after taking on new clients. And who doesn't like easy? That's one of the reasons my program is so incredibly sustainable. The light structure of the Fab Four and the Fab Four Smoothie makes eating to satiety a breeze and allows your body's natural metabolism to go to work for you. But that's not the only reason the plan is so effective and sustainable.

It works because it's **flexible** and **adaptable** to real life. After all, a lifestyle is one you can *actually live,* right? And that's what I coach and guide my clients to do—live! Personally, I like to know I can live spur of the moment if I want to, and not be tied to my home, a strict eating schedule, or an overly restrictive meal plan. I like to know I can change up my meals, my smoothies, and even my shopping routine, all without falling off the wagon. I want the same for you—the ability to live life as it comes, without overthinking every food decision along the way. I want you to feel empowered and in control, no matter the location, setting, or mood you're in.

What follows is a collection of simple tools, tips, and strategies that will help you tackle a variety of real-life what-to-buy/eat/order moments, so you can get in the groove of your very own Fab Four lifestyle. You'll find tips on how to plan meals and shop; how to stay in balance even if you travel for work, let your hair down on a long weekend, or go on vacation; and how to easily regain balance if a night out or #sundayfunday throws you off-kilter. There won't be any menu, party, airport, work conference, or weekend at the in-laws' you can't handle!

Remember, this lifestyle is about nourishing your body, loving yourself, and enjoying the pleasures of life. I've made it my mission to give you simple strategies to find balance and ditch that all-or-nothing diet mentality that might be weighing you down. Within no time, I promise you'll sense a new confidence growing inside you, and this way of thinking will become automatic.

Here you go!

PLAN IN THREE-DAY INCREMENTS

If you usually cook at home, it's natural to want to plan and shop for the entire five- or seven-day week. You might also want (or need) to do as much Sunday meal prep as possible. I'm all for planning and Sunday meal prep, but I don't recommend thinking in weeklong terms. Instead, I coach my clients to think in blocks of no more than three days at a time.

Thinking in three-day increments gives you more flexibility, both mentally and in terms of your actual food decisions. It's probably not realistic to decide on a Sunday what you're going to want to eat by Thursday or Friday. Plus, some aspect of your weekly schedule may have changed by Wednesday—you worked late, had an impromptu dinner out, or just didn't feel like cooking (or eating what you did cook). It makes trips to the grocery store quicker and easier and reduces the amount of time you need to spend doing Sunday meal prep. It also limits waste and ensures that your ingredients are as fresh as possible. In addition, I tend to go out to eat later in the week and on the weekends, which means my second grocery trip is normally supplemental—maybe I buy some more greens for a side salad, fresh almond milk for my smoothies, or eggs for a lazy breakfast-for-dinner. The bottom line is that three-day increments give you the ability to plan and be efficient but offer a more realistic, livable, and flexible time frame.

The effect of this kind of planning is food sanity, not food anxiety. If I have to plan ahead for an entire week, I end up feeling overwhelmed or annoyed, or I turn into a human garbage disposal racing to eat all my prepped food before it goes bad. Have you ever prepped on Sunday and eaten it all by Wednesday, or staggered into Friday with 50 percent of your planned food uneaten?

Many of my clients have had this problem. They've shared with me that trying to think ahead for an entire week reminds them of strict seven-day diets, which can lead to the restrictive, "on or off plan" mentality we're trying to replace. Further, this kind of planning and overstructuring can also trigger food obsession and other negative patterns of thinking. Believe me, I've been there. And I get why many diets offer seven-day meal plans: so people don't have to overthink what they are going to eat. Yes, on the one hand, people like to be told what to do and what to eat. But ultimately, I think our human default mode is freedom! Besides, overplanning meals takes away the pleasure of shopping, preparing, and enjoying them. Three-day increments are the perfect sweet spot and have been highly effective for my clients.

◆

WHERE TO SHOP

I tend to go to stores that offer a wide variety of organic produce, meats, fish, and staple items. Whole Foods and Trader Joe's are my two go-tos, but many other regional and national grocery chains now offer whole, organic, and unprocessed foods. It's a positive trend and it means even places like Costco, Target, and Walmart might be options for you, depending on where you live. (Just do a little research and read all your labels very carefully!)

Have you ever ventured out to a local farmers' market? Many communities and neighborhoods around the country have weekly or monthly farmers' markets where you can find fresh and healthy foods. If I go to the farmers' market on Sunday, I know I can find my organic vegetables, herbs, and some fun new dips and sauces. It's also a great place to buy wild fish, grass-finished beef (which was raised only on pasture, as opposed to grass-fed animals, which are often grain-fed for part of their lives and grass-fed only closer to slaughter), and cage-free eggs and poultry. Talking directly with independent farmers and growers will also give you a different perspective and connect you to where your food comes from.

Obviously, everything is online these days, too. There's no shortage of subscription meal services, shopping apps, and websites out there to choose from. But make sure you take a close look at these options. Sun Basket and Green Chef, for instance, offer many organic, non-GMO choices, whereas more commercial, mainstream services such as Blue Apron offer meals that include a lot of fatty, salty, and sweet sauces and ingredients, and they don't promise that meats and vegetables are organic. When it comes to fresh, organic produce, you can't turn to your former excuses about not having the time to shop. Amazon Fresh, UberEATS, and others make shopping and planning your meals super easy and much less time consuming. I've found that sourcing my proteins on-line has been extremely efficient. It's easy to buy meat, poultry, and fish in bulk and store it my freezer, then just pull out what I need or feel like that week or morning. My favorite online resources include Butcher Box, Vital Choice, Honest Bison, and U.S. Wellness Meats. Local, independent farms may also have online presences. For specialty items that are hard to find, or more expensive shelf-stable ingredients such as coconut aminos, approved protein bars, and individual travel supplies, I like to order online from Thrive Market. Having specialty supplies on hand helps me upgrade my meals, stay on track, and avoid using or eating food that isn't clean.

Tips for Shopping and Light Planning

- **MAKE A LIST BEFORE YOU GO SHOPPING.** As I create a cluster of meals for my three-day increment, I think about how certain meals and their ingredients overlap. I don't like to waste food, so this helps me use all the fresh ingredients on my shopping list and make sure what I need in the staples department is on hand.
- **DON'T SHOP HUNGRY.** You've no doubt heard this tip before, but it's worth another reminder. Going to a grocery store hungry is just plain dangerous! When we're in a state of low blood sugar, we're hormonally driven toward the sweets, treats, and starches. The key is to time your shopping for after a meal or smoothie.
- **GET TO KNOW YOUR LOCAL GROCERY AND FARMERS' MARKET OPTIONS.** Ideally, you want a grocery store with a wide range of organic and unprocessed foods. If you're doing a lot of shopping online, I recommend Thrive Market and Amazon Fresh.

WHAT TO BUY

I tend to shop on Sundays, and when I do, I like to have a loose idea of what I plan to make for lunch and dinner, working off my calendar and knowing when I'll be prepping for two or just for me. As you will see, many of the items on my grocery list are staples—they can be bought more or less in bulk and keep well in your refrigerator, freezer, or cupboard for a month or so. This is why I usually have two grocery lists—one that changes weekly, based on my recipes, meals, and smoothies, and one that includes staples that don't vary all that much from month to month.

I like simple, tasty meals. I purchase things that inspire my appetite and balance my body. Keeping my cabinets stocked with dry, canned, and fridge-stable supplies like chia, flaxseed, coconut milk, garbanzo beans, and nut butters makes it easy to whip up a meal without extra planning. My bulk online protein order guarantees I always have protein and it normally includes: 2 pints of bone broth; 2 to 4 pounds of grass-finished ground beef; 1 or 2 steaks (bison or grass-finished beef); 1 whole chicken; 4 chicken breasts; 1 pound of jumbo wild shrimp; and 4 pieces of wild salmon. If something is on special or looks super yummy—maybe lobster, scallops, whitefish, bacon, or ribs—I simply add it to the cart. I try to cook through the whole order before I order again.

Then, when I do get to the farmers' market, I may need to pick up only one vegetable to roast for each dinner, such as Brussels sprouts, asparagus, broccolini, or cauliflower, depending on what looks fresh and appealing. I also throw in the fixings for a crunchy salad (greens, vegetables, cucumber, tomatoes, and so on), plus an aromatic or two (onions, garlic, and some good-looking herbs). That leaves only avocados, eggs, lemons and limes, and something to keep it fun, like fat sauces such as hummus, chimichurri, baba ghanoush, or pasta sauce. These basics set me up for all my favorite dishes, such as broccolini beef, zoodles and meat sauce, lemon chicken with roasted veggies, lettuce-wrapped burgers, chicken fab pho bowl, or taco night. (Find all these recipes in chapter 6, starting on page 104!)

When your favorites can be whipped up in ten minutes, Sunday prep turns into cleaning veggies, making a bulk protein, a fat sauce, or freezer fudge (see this fave recipe on page 134). And when it comes to Sunday night dinner, we tend to eat a soup I pick up from the farmers' market and a few roasted veggies from my prep.

Here's a version of a play-by-play for your Sunday Fab Four prep:

- **PROTEIN:** Prepare one bulk protein that can be used for lunch, a weeknight dinner, or a post-weight-training bridge snack. You can roast a whole chicken, hard-boil half a carton of eggs, prepare flax meatballs, or whip up a salmon salad.
- **FAT:** Make a fat sauce, such as avocado hummus, chimichurri, pesto, or a salad dressing. If you feel your sweet tooth kicking in, make freezer fudge for the week.
- **FIBER AND GREENS:** Wash and chop salad produce for easy use. Roast two trays of vegetables for sides or cold lunch salads.
- **HERBS:** Freeze half your herbs for smoothies or recipes (see sidebar, page 186).
- **SUPER SUNDAY EXTRAS:** If you have time, make a chili, soup, or puree that you love.

Smoothie supplies are the easiest to keep on hand, making it really simple to eat clean and balance your blood sugar. Protein powders, chia, flaxseeds, acacia fiber, coconut milk, cacao nibs, adaptogens, shredded coconut, hemp hearts, walnuts, MCT oil, and coconut oil are all shelf-stable, so no excuses! Plus, nut butters last in the fridge and unopened backups can be stored in the pantry. Then you can load up your freezer with frozen spinach, kale, berries, and a seasonal fruit to experiment with in a new recipe. What tends to work for my clients is finding a few staple recipes for smoothies and then trying a new one once a week or so.

Smoothies can help you use up your farmers' market leftovers, too. For example, squeeze a leftover half lemon into your smoothie for phytonutrients, and don't forget to throw in those fresh herbs, cucumbers, and greens before they wilt.

Sunday Fab Four Smoothie checklist: Ensure you have protein, fat, fiber, and a liquid source for a week of smoothies. Unlike meal planning, smoothie planning should get you through a week of breakfast smoothies.

Buy organic nuts in bulk, keep them in the freezer to prevent oxidation, and portion out what you need into a glass container for the week.

MY "STAPLES" GROCERY LIST

While "staples" traditionally refers simply to dry goods that can be stored in your cupboard, for our purposes the idea of staples includes all the regular, clean foods that you will be incorporating into your smoothies and Fab Four meals. Here's my list of grocery staples:

For Your Freezer

Soup: bone broth, bulk vegetable soup, homemade chili

Seafood: wild fish, salmon, halibut, shrimp, sole, scallops

Red meat: grass-finished bison, beef, and lamb; premade flax-meal meatballs

Poultry: organic free-range chicken and turkey breasts

Organic frozen berries

Organic frozen vegetables and greens

For Your Fridge

Homemade fat sauces: pesto, chimichurri, guacamole

Prepared protein: turkey slices, grass-finished beef meatballs, roasted whole chicken

Salad greens: one staple (romaine, spinach, or mixed greens) and one "push" (microgreens, red-leaf lettuce, chard . . .)

Prepped veggies: containers of fresh veggies, washed and cut up

Eggs: cage-free, hard-boiled

Condiments and Oils

Hot sauce: Organicville gluten-free Sky Valley Sriracha Sauce, Tapatio, Cholula

Nut butters: organic almond, pecan, walnut, macadamia, and cashew

Guacamole

Fresh salsa

Mustard: Dijon, yellow

Coconut aminos (This is a soy sauce alternative—gluten-free with a fifth of the sodium!)

Avocado oil mayonnaise: Primal Kitchen mayonnaise

Homemade Hummus (page 125) or Avocado Hummus (page 125)

For Your Pantry

Nuts: Choose from the bulk raw almonds, cashews, pecans, walnuts, macadamia, Brazil nuts, pistachios. (Keep no more than a month's worth in your pantry. If you buy a big batch from Costco or another super store, store them in your freezer.)

Dark chocolate: soy- and dairy-free—some of my favorite organic brands are Theo, Eating Evolved, and Hu

Tetra Pak (aseptic) cartons or BPA-free cans: organic beans, broths, nut or coconut milk

Black bean chips: higher in fiber than corn chips

Flax crackers: such as Mary's Gone Crackers and Jilz Crackers

Wraps: Paleo coconut wraps, raw dehydrated wraps, rice paper wraps, and Seite tortillas

Gluten-free starch: ancient black rice, California-grown rice, quinoa

Dried spices and herbs: Remember, organic when possible!

    Basil

    Cilantro (fresh)

Chili powder

Cocoa powder (unsweetened)

Cayenne

Cumin

Herbes de Provence

Rosemary (fresh and dried)

Oregano

Parsley

Black pepper

Pink Himalayan salt

Red pepper flakes

Smoked paprika

Thyme (fresh and dried)

MAKING BODY-LOVING CHOICES

When selecting foods that fit your Fab Four or Fab Four Smoothie formula, choose sources with the most nutritional value. Here's a quick guide to the best choices for fat, carbohydrates (greens as well as starchy carbs), fiber, and proteins. As always, it's better to go organic when possible!

Optimal Fat Choices

Algae oil

Avocado

Avocado oil

Coconut milk

Coconut oil

Cultured or pastured organic butter

Flaxseed oil

Freshly ground flaxseed meal

Ghee (pasture-raised butter or grass-fed ghee)

QUICK SEASONINGS

Store these in your pantry and you're ready to go! If you enjoy salt,
add a pinch to those mixes that don't require it.

CHILI MIX

2 tablespoons chili powder

$^1/_2$ tablespoon smoked paprika

$^1/_2$ teaspoon dried oregano

$^1/_2$ teaspoon cayenne

$^1/_2$ teaspoon ground cumin

$^1/_2$ teaspoon freshly ground black
  pepper

1 teaspoon pink Himalayan salt

TACO MIX

1 tablespoon chili powder

$1^1/_2$ teaspoons paprika (smoked
  optional)

$1^1/_2$ teaspoons ground cumin

$1^1/_2$ teaspoons garlic powder

$1^1/_2$ teaspoons onion powder

$^3/_4$ to $1^1/_2$ teaspoons red pepper flakes

ITALIAN MIX

1 teaspoon dried oregano

1 teaspoon dried basil

1 teaspoon dried rosemary

1 teaspoon dried thyme

1 teaspoon dried sage

MEDITERRANEAN MIX

3 tablespoons parsley flakes

3 tablespoons dried thyme

3 tablespoons dried oregano

1 to $1^1/_2$ tablespoons dried basil
  leaves

1 to $1^1/_2$ tablespoons dried grated
  lemon peel

$^1/_2$ teaspoon celery seed

GARLIC AND HERB MIX

2 tablespoons dried oregano

2 tablespoons dried basil

2 tablespoons parsley flakes

1 tablespoon onion powder

1 tablespoon ground thyme

1 tablespoon pink Himalayan salt

2 teaspoons garlic powder

1 teaspoon freshly ground black
  pepper

Olive oil (extra-virgin if used in
   salads)

Olives

Raw nuts: bulk raw almonds, cashews,
   pecans, walnuts, macadamia nuts,
   Brazil nuts, pistachios

Body-Loving Nonstarchy Vegetables

Artichokes	Fennel
Arugula	Garlic
Asparagus	Green beans
Bamboo shoots	Jalapeños
Bean sprouts	Jicama
Beet greens	Kale
Bell peppers (red, yellow, green)	Kohlrabi
Broccoli	Leeks
Brussels sprouts	Lettuce
Cabbage	Mushrooms
Carrots	Mustard greens
Cassava	Onions
Cauliflower	Parsley
Celery	Pumpkin
Chicory	Radicchio
Chives	Radishes
Cilantro	Shallots
Collard greens	Spinach
Cucumber	Squash (acorn, butternut, spaghetti, summer, winter)
Dandelion greens	
Eggplant	Swiss chard
Endive	Tomatoes

Turnips
Turnip greens

Watercress
Zucchini

Body-Loving Legume Options

Black beans
Cannellini (white) beans
Chickpeas (garbanzo beans)
Kidney beans

Lentils
Navy beans
Pinto beans
Peanuts

Body-Loving High-Fiber, Non-Starchy Carbohydrate Choices

Zoodles
Cauliflower Rice

Homemade cauliflower pizza crust

Body-Loving High-Fiber, Starchy Carbohydrate Choices

Quinoa
California basmati rice, California wild rice, brown rice, or sushi rice

Gluten-free pasta (one or two times per month)
Sweet potatoes or yams
Tortillas, grain free or organic corn

Body-Loving Daily Fruit Choices

Blackberries
Blueberries
Boysenberries
Raspberries

Strawberries
½ apple
Lemon
Lime

Body-Loving Weekly Fruit Choices (enjoy these sweet fruits only once or twice a week)

Apples	Passion fruit
Bananas	Peaches
Cherries	Pears
Fresh apricots	Persimmons
Grapefruits	Plums
Kiwis	Pomegranates
Melons	Tangerines
Nectarines	Watermelon
Oranges	

Body-Loving Monthly Produce Choices (these fruits and veggies have a high impact on your blood sugar, so enjoy them sparingly)

Corn	Peas
Dates	Pineapples
Dried fruits	White potatoes
Grapes	

TIP: If the herbs you have on hand don't easily mix into your smoothie flavor that day, you can: chop and then freeze them in an ice cube tray with a little coconut, ghee, or olive oil for a future recipe; freeze them in an ice cube tray with water for a future smoothie; or blend them into a pesto, hummus, dip, or sauce to use within 3 to 5 days.

◆

SIMPLE SUBSTITUTIONS

Much of the success and ease of the Fab Four lifestyle comes from making simple, healthy, and delicious substitutions that can have a dramatic impact on your health. Initially, these replacements might take you a little out of your comfort zone, but I encourage you to embrace being in unfamiliar territory and try them out. In a few short weeks, you might just find yourself with an expanded palate. The upside is huge—improved overall health, new flavors, flexibility if you're facing a challenging menu or situation, and confidence in a new growth-oriented mind-set.

Instead of Beef . . . Try Buffalo (Bison) or Lamb

Yearning for a big burger, guilt-free steak, or tasty bowl of chili? Try swapping buffalo (bison) for your conventionally raised beef or chicken. Lower in cholesterol and fat than chicken and higher in protein than beef, buffalo is becoming a popular substitute. It contains zinc and selenium, two must-have minerals for thyroid health, it's loaded with magnesium and potassium, and it offers essential amino acids our bodies can't produce on their own, like lysine. Lamb is a high-quality protein source that is also rich in micronutrients, such as iron, zinc, and vitamin B12.

Instead of Table Salt . . . Try Pink Himalayan Salt

Ditch your table salt! Pink Himalayan salt is packed with more than eighty-four trace minerals and elements, as opposed to table salt, which is 97.5 percent sodium chloride with an anticaking agent (not good!). Excess sodium chloride increases your risk of hypertension, osteoporosis, and kidney disease, whereas the diversity of elements in pink Himalayan salt creates an electrolyte balance within your body, strengthens bones, lowers blood pressure, and improves circulation. It also helps you protect the delicate balance of minerals in your cells, avoid excess water retention, and prevent premature aging. Processed foods are loaded with sodium chloride, so limit your processed food intake, and when cooking at home, use some of the less-processed choices, including kosher salt, sea salt, and of course, the pink stuff—it tastes amazing!

Instead of Soy Sauce or Tamari . . . Try Coconut Aminos

This is one of my personal favorites. Swapping coconut aminos for both soy sauce and tamari has a number of clean benefits. Coconut aminos are made from coconut sap and natural sea salt. This salty replacement contains seventeen amino acids and B vitamins, and ditching soy means eliminating phytoestrogens, phytic acid, and MSG (monosodium glutamate), all of which are bad for you. It also means consuming 700 milligrams *less* sodium than you otherwise would if using soy sauce or tamari. That's the difference between 36 percent of your daily recommended sodium intake and a mere 5 percent. Bloaty sushi hangover, begone!

Instead of Swordfish . . . Try Salmon, Tuna, or Sardines

Canned cold-water fish (such as tuna, herring, salmon, mackerel, or sardines) are a great source of protein and healthy omega-3 fat. However, some have gotten a bad rap due to their mercury content. Mercury is a neurotoxin that interferes with the brain and nervous system, fertility, and fetal development. The good news is selenium binds to mercury and prevents it from creating mercury toxicity in your body, so as long as the fish you're eating contains more selenium than mercury, you don't need to worry. Unfortunately, that means swordfish is out, but you don't have to avoid tuna altogether. My suggestion is to mix it up and go for the richest sources of omega-3. Two of the most delicious are salmon and sardines. Sardines are one of the most concentrated sources of the omega-3 fatty acids EPA and DHA, and provide three times your daily recommended vitamin B12. If you find it hard to stomach sardines, salmon is a great option to hydrate your cells with omega-3s while lowering your "bad" triglycerides and cholesterol levels.

Instead of Cheese Made from Cow's Milk . . . Try Goat's, Sheep's, or Nut Milk Cheese

Cow dairy (unless organic and 100 percent grass-fed) contains antibiotics and growth factors that are intended to grow baby cows, not humans! Regular consumption of cow dairy can result in IBS and may exacerbate asthma, other respiratory and sinus disorders, and some skin conditions. Goat's and sheep's milk cheeses are two delicious swaps that don't come with all that potential baggage; plus, they are lower in lactose. Fermented nut milk cheese (such as the almond cream cheese substitute from Kite Hill) is a great way to get a little protein, good bacteria, and cheesy flavor without the dairy. It may sound a little different, but trust me—even my cheddar-loving husband digs it!

Instead of Rice . . . Try Amaranth, Millet, or Quinoa

In 2012, an article in *Consumer Reports* revealed that there are unsafe levels of arsenic in more than sixty varieties of rice! A subsequent article in 2014 reconfirmed these findings by testing an additional 128 samples. Arsenic is linked to an increased risk of bladder, lung, and skin cancer. It accumulates in the outer layers of rice, which are removed to make white rice. As a result, brown rice may contain 80 percent more arsenic than the white varieties. Furthermore, arsenic levels may vary by region and types of rice. White basmati rice from California and sushi rice have 38 percent *less* arsenic than white rice from Arkansas, Texas, and Louisiana, which offer among the highest levels. So save your rice for sushi nights and pick up a clean California-grown rice for your home. Alternative grains to rice such as amaranth, millet, and quinoa all contain significantly less arsenic than rice. These "ancient," non-GMO options are also rich in fiber.

Instead of Conventional Wine . . . Try Organic Wine

Natural, organic, and biodynamic wine is the way to go if you like your vino. These are free of added sulfites, fructose, and pesticides. Sulfites are naturally occurring in wine, but nowadays they're added in large quantities to enhance flavor, complexity, and depth. Choose wine without added sulfites when you can, because those compounds are what cause broken capillaries, sinus mucus, headaches, swelling, sneezing, rashes, and acne. Furthermore, the dirty little secret of wine makers is the addition of a high-fructose grape juice concentrate called "mega purple" to increase palatability—but it also increases your waistline. And do I need to explain why you shouldn't drink pesticides? (wink) Looking for a good source of organic wine? Check out www.dryfarmwines.com.

Instead of Cream in Your Coffee . . . Add Coconut Oil, Coconut Milk, or Nut Milk

If you're looking to avoid cow dairy (you should!), but still love a frothy latte, blend 1 tablespoon of coconut oil (or milk) into a cup of hot coffee or tea. Coconut oil contains lots of healthy fat that can help kick-start your metabolism in the morning. When blended, the fat emulsifies into a creamy latte consistency (thanks, Dave!). The coconut flavor won't overpower the coffee; it will add just the slightest hint of sweetness. If you opt for a nut milk latte, make it unsweetened. Sadly, Starbucks coconut milk doesn't count.

Here are some other quick-fire swaps to try out:

- **INSTEAD OF WHITE POTATOES . . . TRY PARSNIPS AND CAULIFLOWER.** Mashed or roasted, they make a great, less starchy replacement that will still fill you up.
- **INSTEAD OF WHEAT PASTA . . . TRY ZOODLES (SEE PAGE 106) AND SPAGHETTI SQUASH.** These are delicious veggie replacements for starchy pasta noodles. You add taste and fiber to your noodle dish while avoiding gluten and nonfibrous carbohydrates. Save the pasta night for an anniversary dinner, a European vacation, or your mom's famous holiday lasagna (and remember that pasta servings in Italy are much smaller than the usual American carb-fest!).
- **INSTEAD OF CRACKERS WITH YOUR DIPS . . . TRY RADISH SLICES OR CUCUMBER, BELL PEPPER, OR PARSNIP STICKS.** This will help cut down on sodium, carbohydrates, and sugar. They'll also fill you up due to water content and fiber, helping you to eat less overall.
- **INSTEAD OF REGULAR MAYONNAISE . . . TRY AVOCADO OIL MAYONNAISE.** It adds great texture and flavor in chicken, salmon, and tuna salad.
- **INSTEAD OF REGULAR EGGS . . . TRY ORGANIC, CAGE-FREE, AND OMEGA-3 EGGS.** Always! The chickens are fed flax and their eggs provide us with an anti-inflammatory boost!
- **INSTEAD OF REGULAR CRACKERS . . . TRY HIGH FIBER CRACKERS MADE WITH CHIA AND FLAX.** They lower your glucose response and increase daily fiber intake.
- **INSTEAD OF REGULAR HUMMUS . . . TRY BLENDING YOUR OWN AND LIGHTENING IT UP WITH VEGETABLES.** Mix in spinach, zucchini, or avocado to lighten it up while adding fat, fiber, and greens.

MEAL PREP HACKS

I understand that some of you don't have the time, inclination, or interest to cook at home on a daily basis. And while I promise you that the recipes you'll find in chapter 6 are really easy (!), I get it—we all enjoy going to lunch, brunch, and dinner with friends and colleagues. We can all get stuck in schedules of long hours and too little time or energy at the end of the day to delight in making a meal. So, with that in mind, here's a list of my favorite hacks for eating in situations where you might have less control.

- Create an inventory of takeout or delivery menus from establishments serving clean food, so when you get hungry, you have good choices at the ready.
- Keep lists of the local restaurants in various categories (different cuisines and expense levels) where you have clean-eating options.
- If your friends are gathering at a place that might put you off the rails, use a Fab Four Smoothie to balance your blood sugar in advance. You'll be able to order something simple from the appetizer menu without going hungry.
- Become familiar with my recipes that integrate premade food, like dishes that include an organic rotisserie chicken you can pick up at the store. You can quickly build a chicken teriyaki bowl with your already-prepared protein. The same goes if you want to make takeout sushi a Fab Four meal: pick up some hamachi crudo at your favorite grocery store, add avocado and grapefruit slices, and drizzle with a fave fat sauce. It's an instant Fab Four meal!

What's the takeaway here? Again, you're relying on **light structure** in your approach to eating so that you can enjoy food without getting too restrictive!

BEWARE OF THESE ITEMS!

SEED OILS

Almost exclusively omega-6, these oils have replaced a number of trans fats over the last decade. Eating an excessive amount of omega-6 disrupts the balance of omegas in your body and will lead to increased inflammation. Try your best to avoid sauces, dressings, and foods that contain the following oils: safflower, sunflower, corn, soybean, cottonseed, grapeseed, and canola. Read your food labels!

PARABENS

These chemical preservatives have been on lists of what to avoid in beauty products for years, but food labels remain somewhat of an uncharted territory. Sure, if you're a clean-eating, whole-food-devoted health nut who avoids all processed foods, food labels don't even concern you, but most of us often encounter unknown ingredients on food labels. So continue to eat clean as much as you can, stock up on healthy essentials like organic coconut oil and raw apple cider vinegar, and avoid these preservatives when grocery shopping. They're very unnatural sounding words on food labels with "E-numbers" and ingredient that contains the word *paraben*, such as methylparaben (E218), ethylparaben (E214), propylparaben (E216), heptylparaben (E209), and butylparaben.

ISOFLAVONES

Isoflavones are estrogen-like compounds found in such foods as peanuts, chickpeas, alfalfa sprouts, fava beans, and soy foods that can cause reproductive problems, weight gain, and fatigue. In the small naturally occurring quantities of peanuts, chickpeas, alphalfa sprouts and fava beans, there is nothing to worry about. Soy products on the other hand can contain 10–60 times the isoflavone quantity of those foods. Research has shown that isoflavones in large quantities can prevent ovulation and stimulate cancerous cell growth. Not only is soy potentially harmful to your reproductive system, it's also not great for your skin. It's full of phytoestrogens that can cause breakouts and hormonal blemishes around the mouth and jawline. I am pretty particular about this one—soy is not a health food!

BPA AND BPO

Harmful chemicals can still be found hiding in BPA-free plastics, since some manufacturers have simply replaced BPA with BPO. These chemicals bind to the estrogen that is naturally occurring in the body and, in effect, increase the amount of estrogen in the bloodstream. Medical research suggests that an increase in estrogen can interfere with your libido and reproductive organs and even result in weight gain. Heat and sunlight on plastic water bottles exacerbate the negative effects of these chemicals, so think twice before leaving a water bottle to bake in your car. Or better yet, opt for reusable glass bottles to avoid these harmful effects.

MONOSODIUM GLUTAMATE (MSG)

This additive in processed and fast foods is meant to add flavor, but in reality it just masks the true taste of the food! MSG is a manufactured chemical made in part from the amino acid glutamic acid and acts as a contaminant on the body. Glutamate is essential for cognitive function. It acts as a stimulant and signals the messengers in our brain cells to communicate. However, free-bound glutamate ingested in abundance, such as in food with added MSG, can overexcite the nervous system and cause headaches, migraines, and inflammation. The best way to avoid MSG is to shop the perimeter of the grocery store and avoid any prepackaged, extra-salty snacks, but if you do shop those inner aisles, check the labels and avoid this unnecessary ingredient!

CARRAGEENAN

Carrageenan can be found in both almond and coconut milk and is often used as a food thickener or stabilizer. Studies suggest that an increase in exposure to carrageenan can cause intestinal inflammation and lead to digestive problems. While the harmful evidence is not overwhelming (yet), it's best to avoid carrageenan and double-check the label when buying nondairy nut milk.

GUAR GUM

A by-product of the guar bean, guar gum has raised concern due to its prevalence in canned coconut milk. Studies report that consuming guar gum may result in gastrointestinal side effects such as increased gas and abdominal discomfort. If you have digestive issues, removing guar gum from your diet may improve these symptoms.

STAYING WELL ON THE ROAD . . . NEAR AND FAR

Travel of any kind can pose a challenge to our diets. Long drives and road trips are full of convenient temptation—fast-food signs, gas station snacks, greasy diners—with healthy options seldom to be found. Work trips and conferences usually entail airports, train stations, dinners and drinks with colleagues, and access to hotel minibars and vending machines. Vacations present their own quandaries. Whether you're traveling domestic or international, you may not have access to a kitchen or the types of clean, organic grocery stores and restaurants you're used to at home. And when you're in vacay mode, the temptation to cut loose and go binge might be hard to resist. Here are some tips that will help keep you in balance without making you crazy. And remember, as soon as you are home, you know how to autocorrect so you'll be back on track in no time.

START TRAVEL DAYS WITH A FULL BELLY. I try to start any travel day with a full belly. If you leave home hungry, it can be just too tempting to grab junk or fast food as you run through the airport or at a rest stop. Eating poorly at the beginning of the trip can set you up for days of bad eating, so prepare for day one appropriately. My favorite pre-travel breakfast at home is the Spa Day Smoothie (page 142), loaded with extra greens and half an avocado. If you know your airport has restaurants that offer clean meals for lunch and dinner, then by all means, go for it. LAX, my hometown airport, has recently added some reliable options. But remember, you want to create the closest mix of the Fab Four formula—protein, fat, fiber, and greens. Another option is to leave home a bit early and drop by your local grocery store to pick up a clean meal at the salad bar, hot bar, or deli that you know will taste good and fill you up on your flight.

On the way home, I try to eat a satisfying Fab Four meal, such as a veggie omelet with avocado or a salmon salad. If you've indulged yourself on a trip, you can be tempted to jump into deprivation mode, but that's a mistake—odds are that when you finally walk in the front door, you'll be tired and hangry, craving sugary, high-carbohydrate comfort foods. As with any other day, the key is to start your body with enough protein, fat, and fiber to hold you over between meals and keep your blood sugar balanced.

HAVE GOOD TRAVEL SNACKS HANDY. As I mentioned earlier, I prefer eating filling meals over quick-fix snacks, and generally advise my clients not to make snacks their go-to travel meal option. Snacks can be little triggers of temptation that can set off a blood sugar spike and inevitable crash. Remember that crazy up-and-down cycle we are trying to flatten out? Snacks tend to interrupt that peaceful wave we are trying to create.

All that said, travel can sometimes throw you out of whack through no fault of your own, so I do recommend that you travel prepared with a few approved snacks. My go-to flight or driving snacks are hard-boiled eggs, nut packs, almond butter packs with celery slices, or a bag of sliced or diced water-rich veggies, such as cucumbers. I also bring protein powder packets and a shake bottle. In fact, I never leave home without my to-go Fab Four Smoothie kit! (See the sidebar on page 198 for details.) It's so easy to snag an iced coffee or tea and shake it with some protein to help bridge me to my next meal.

EATING OUT. Traveling typically entails eating out at restaurants. So how do you manage that a few days in a row? I start my day with either a smoothie or an almond or coconut butter travel pack from Artisana (no added sugar or palm oil), or if the breakfast looks exceptionally delicious, I enjoy eggs from a buffet. Depending on how hungry I am, I make lunch a salad with as many crunchy vegetables as possible. But again, you need to include a healthy fat with your salad—a side of avocado, olives, nuts, or a clean dressing.

I find dinners fairly easy, usually because there is more to choose from. I always select an entrée that features a protein—grilled fish or red meat that I know is local and/or organic. I watch the sides, as they are often full of starchy carbohydrates, and if possible, I pair the protein with at least two vegetables, such as a mixed salad and roasted veggies.

If you're staying in one location for more than three or four days, you can do some light homework. If possible (and language barriers are not a problem), choose at least one restaurant that offers you clean food dishes. You might also check out travel or food bloggers covering the area. I've found awesome restaurants that offer delicious clean-food and gluten-free dishes. The last time I was in Rome, I was even able to find a gluten-free pasta bar!

The best strategy for keeping yourself on an even keel while traveling

TRAVEL CHECKLIST

1. **SMOOTHIE:** protein packets (1.5 per day), a shaker bottle, and a zip-top bag of chia seeds

2. **MINI FAT PACKS:** nut butters, coconut butter, and coconut oil

3. **BRIDGE SNACKS:** individual nut packs, chopped veggies, and approved bars (Bulletproof or Primal Kitchen)

4. **SLEEP:** earplugs, eye mask, and lavender essential oil

5. **SKIN:** calendula oil, lip balm, and hydration spray

is simply making clean-food choices when you're in a restaurant that you have not researched beforehand: instead of fried dishes, choose grilled; instead of sautéed veggies, ask to have them steamed or grilled. In my experience, you can make these polite requests in any language!

If you're poolside on vacation, politely ask for some simple swaps. If they're serving guac with chips, ask for crudités instead; if you'd love the burger, ask for it to be wrapped in lettuce or to come without the bun. When it comes to room service, the same swap mentality can apply. You can also ask them to skip the morning bread basket, jellies, or even ketchup.

What happens if your travels take you to someone's home, such as your in-laws' or your great-aunt Marguerite's? First, remember that family is family, so you should feel empowered to tell them what you eat and don't eat. But be proactive and offer to bring a salad, clean entrée, or veggie side. This is a polite gesture that signals you are taking care of yourself and not burdening them unduly—and who knows, they may love the food and want to know more about your clean-eating lifestyle!

TREAT YOURSELF . . . BUT WISELY. While on vacation, don't be afraid to enjoy yourself. That's the point! Vacation is a time for decompressing, recharging, and living outside your usual life. If you're in a foreign country, kick back and enjoy the specialties of the area—in Italy, gelato; in France, *pain au chocolat*; or in Mexico, fresh tortilla chips and guacamole! These indulgences are good for the soul, but if you don't want to come home feeling bloated, irritable, and heavier, then there are ways to keep yourself in balance even while relaxing. On vacation, my favorite indulgence is wine or a cocktail. When I have a drink or two, I pass on dessert. It's about making wise choices in the moment and savoring what you do choose. Remember that if you're living in a restrictive diet mentality, you are much more likely to go off-plan completely. Excuses such as "I'll eat whatever I want today and start the diet tomorrow" just set you up to crave and cave. Think of treats as either satisfying tastes that you enjoy or a glass of something special to relax you.

MOVE YOUR BODY. On vacation, I also try to include some exercise or movement every day. If I'm touring, that means walking instead of taking a taxi. If I'm at a resort, I swim, sign up for a fitness class, or hit the gym on my own. If I'm at the beach, I take a long walk or run in the sand. I'm not super strict, but I know that I feel better when I break a sweat and get even 20 to 30 minutes of exercise every day. Vacation is my downtime, but it's also about doing what I love, which includes moving my body! (See page 208 for more ways to integrate exercise into your daily life.)

HAVE YOUR FUN . . . WITHOUT LOSING YOUR BALANCE: PLANNING FOR PARTIES AND HOLIDAYS

Making it through a party or a long holiday season without a little indulgence is practically impossible. The best way to stay balanced and still enjoy yourself is by getting used to a few strategies.

PLAY DETECTIVE. How many times do you check ingredients and menus before a work lunch? Being similarly prepared for a party or event allows you to make decisions ahead of time and stick to your guns. So ask some questions. Will there be a full meal or passed appetizers only? Will there be beer and wine or a full bar? Is it a potluck? If so, you're in luck! Bring a guilt-free plate, such as a sharable green salad, chicken skewers with coconut aminos, or veggie crudités.

THE PRE-PARTY SMOOTHIE (AKA THE "ROADIE"). Arrive at parties feeling balanced by ingesting 15 to 20 grams of protein in a Fab Four Smoothie before the party. Protein and fat help to balance blood sugar and make us feel satiated. This strategy helps you not to feel ravenous, so you don't grab the first deep-fried appetizer without thinking. My clients affectionately coined this technique the "Roadie" and enjoy a light protein smoothie on the way to their events. It works for showers, weddings, and work dinners, as well as press events, red carpets, and galas. Arriving with balanced blood sugar allows you to feel calm, so you can avoid the holiday party pitfalls or sugar-laden desserts and appetizers.

COMMIT TO A GAME PLAN. Devising a plan allows you to relax and enjoy the company of friends or colleagues. If you have a hard time committing, write your plan down in your Fab Four Notebook before you go, or let a friend know your plan. Dr. Gail Matthews, a psychology professor at Dominican University in California, did a study on goal setting with 267 participants. She found that you are 42 percent more likely to achieve your goals just by writing them down. So how do you figure out your game plan? In advance, decide what you know will make you comfortable. If you're going to a wedding or party, maybe you commit to one no-sugar cocktail, one plate of food, and one clean piece of dark chocolate. Deciding in advance will help you pass on the hors d'oeuvre tray or endless buffet. If the party or gathering is at a restaurant, take a look at the menu online before you go—that way you can decide on what you're going to eat . . . and not go off course if someone else chooses to eat less clean.

EARN YOUR ALCOHOL. Make a pact with yourself that you will work out the day of the event and the day after. A little hangover can throw you off your game and get you out of your healthy routine. The perfect time to work out would be two to three hours before the event, followed by hair and makeup and a Roadie if needed. If you don't have time to work out right before the event, no sweat; just try before work or midday. It is all about staying active and making room in your muscles to suck up the extra holiday glucose.

LIMIT LIBATIONS. The easiest way to hydrate and take a deep breath is to make your first drink alcohol-free. Grab a soda water with lemon or a flat water right when you get there. This technique allows you to work through your first few party jitters without sucking down a cocktail too quickly. It is also nice to survey the party and recommit to your game plan; you might even decide that you don't want to drink at this party. Starting with water is also sometimes easier than trying to put the wine down. Find what works for you. A sparkling water intermission is also a good strategy (throw in a lemon or a lime to give it some flavor).

APPROPRIATE APPETIZERS. Appetizers can quickly add up to a full meal, and some fried options can be a real starch bomb. If you know you'll enjoy the main course, politely decline the small morsels; if you had your Roadie, this should be a cakewalk. However, if you are in need of a little sustenance, go for a protein-based appetizer. The best options include anything that belongs on a seafood tower, a mini lamb chop, or a chicken skewer. The veggie tray and hummus can be a great option—just don't overdo it. Avoid fried food, quiche, and flatbread, which spike blood sugar and contribute to insulin resistance, inflammation, and weight gain. If the appetizers are set up on a table, grab a small plate and fill it once. Remember—you are there to spend time with friends, network, or celebrate, so try to enjoy the conversation instead of the crab cakes.

DESSERT . . . OR DON'T. As I mentioned earlier, I suggest that you make a choice between alcohol and dessert so you don't compound your blood sugar. But that doesn't mean forgoing pleasure. Many of my clients are actually surprised when I tell them that a small piece of dark chocolate is a better option than a fruit plate. Partygoers who choose fruit allow themselves a pretty large portion when one bite of chocolate would hit the spot without the added fructose. Unfortunately, 100 percent of fructose is metabolized in the liver, and with alcohol and fructose both filtering there, we are taxing the body with heavy post-party detoxification duties. Since you don't know if chocolate will be offered, keep a small piece in your fridge or some freezer fudge (page 134) at home. Just knowing you can indulge later will keep you motivated to pass on the added sugar at the party.

DO WHAT'S RIGHT FOR YOU. Many times we eat out of anxiety, habit, or politeness. We end up swallowing foods that don't agree with us or give us food guilt, or worse, we eat foods we don't even like! I recommend that you remember what you love and politely decline what doesn't agree with you. This takes practice, but it always helps to be the first to respond. Make eye contact with the server and politely decline so you don't jump on the band-wagon with everyone else.

Avoid making excuses about why you aren't eating the crab cake or cupcake. You don't owe anyone a justification or an explanation about why you prefer not to eat gluten or dairy, and you certainly don't have to manufacture an intolerance or celiac diagnosis, for instance. "No" is a complete sentence! Unfortunately, however, everyone these days seems to have a lot to say about how and what people eat . . . or choose not to eat. In these situations, simply smile, remark that eating in this way makes you feel better, and change the topic.

AVOIDING HANGOVERS

love a glass of wine to relax and have fun. I don't want to deprive you of your wine, beer, or cocktails. Nor do I want you unable to move or needing a breakfast burrito when you wake up. Here are some tips for you to enjoy yourself without triggering that hateful, hurtful hangover.

1. **HYDRATE BEFORE YOU GO OUT.** Hangovers are caused by dehydration—alcohol acts as a diuretic on your body, taking away fluid. So before you head out for the evening, give your body a lot of fluid. Drink several glasses of water, or better yet, hydrate up with a Fab Four Smoothie!

2. **EAT BEFORE YOU GO OUT.** Just as when I travel, I like to eat before an evening of revelry. I have a smoothie or Fab Four meal so I get into balanced blood sugar, with enough fat and protein to sustain me. Having this in your system will help keep you from spiking and crashing from the sugar in alcohol, and will help to break down acetaldehyde, one of the culprits behind a hangover.

3. **CHOOSE CLEAR AND NATURALLY SUGAR-FREE (NOT "DIET") BEVERAGES AS MUCH AS POSSIBLE.** Dark-colored drinks such as bourbon, whiskey, and fruit-laden mixtures have more chemical compounds called congeners (chemical by-products of alcohol fermentation process) than their light-colored cousins, such as tequila or vodka. Aging substances in darker alcohols include small amounts of chemicals such as methanol, acetone, acetaldehyde, esters, tannins, and aldehydes. Red wine contains tannins, compounds that can trigger headaches for some women and men. Malt liquors, such as whiskey, can trigger hangovers that tend to be more intense.

4. **BOOST YOUR VITAMINS.** Consider drinking an electrolyte-vitamin drink (like Oxylent or 8G) or taking a pre/post drinking supplement to support your body to naturally detoxify (Charcoal Pills, Flyby or DrinkSmart). (I *don't* recommend sugary sports drinks.) Drinking depletes your level of glutathione, which is a naturally occurring antioxidant and cell protector that aids the body's ability to defend against alcohol's toxins. Certain studies point to a

combination of vitamin C plus vitamin B (along with specific amino acids and glucose) to boost your glutathione levels. This might be the year to get your glutathione levels checked—if that's your hangover culprit, why suffer more than you have to?

5. **SWEAT IT OUT OR SLEEP IT OFF.** Working out might release endorphins and make you feel better about your alcohol indulgences, but sweating can make dehydration worse. If you're really "feeling it," sleeping it off can actually be a healthier choice. But I understand needing to move, so if you do opt to work out, aim to drink at least 24 ounces of water per hour.

9

VIBRANCY

YOU KNOW THAT FRIEND who walks into a party and is just glowing? It's not her clothes, the shape of her body, or who she's with that captivates you. It's *her*. Her being, her energy. You might find yourself staring, soaking in the almost tangible good vibes that are beaming out of her. She's the woman who seems lit from within, emanating a bright shimmer that not only attracts others, but gives the entire room a boost of positive energy and a sense of well-being. She's magnetic, and her energy is infectious.

That, my friends, is the quality of vibrancy—a sense of inner vitality and positive, healthy energy. The Chinese call this life force, or aliveness, chi. It's that certain something, or je ne sais quoi, that emerges from taking care of ourselves physically, emotionally, and spiritually. One of the goals of the Fab

Four lifestyle is to stoke your inner vitality and vibrancy. As your body adapts to the balance of blood sugar, your hormones stabilize, and your metabolism begins to settle into a rhythm that keeps your energy level throughout the day, you will naturally begin to nurture an inner brightness of your own. It's one of the amazing results of finding or rediscovering body equilibrium.

I can still remember those days when I felt like I was always fighting not to eat and was restricting my meals. I was constantly hungry and never stopped thinking about food. I was always on some diet or just finishing a diet. When I stopped fighting my body, everyone noticed! My family and friends couldn't believe how much more energy I had—they said I glowed! It was an awesome feeling not to be so distracted by food anymore.

In this chapter, you're going to learn how you can add other lifestyle factors to amp up your chi and stoke this inner fire of vitality!

RETHINKING STRESS

If there's one way to kill that glow, it's with stress. Stress comes from everywhere—work, relationships, health, family, finances, traffic. It racks our nerves, creates anxiety and worry, and ultimately robs us of our energy. The good news is that when we actively learn to manage our stress, we can actually use it as a way to prime our attention, focus our energy, and even revitalize ourselves. It may seem counterintuitive, but you've felt it before—the weight lifts, the road ahead clears, and your anxiety fades in the rearview mirror. You show up at that party and *you're* that girl—the one emanating positivity, the bolt of lightning. By proactively managing stress, you convert it into breakthroughs, victories, and growth. That's how you get your glow back—success over stress.

To be honest, managing your stress is your only option. It's not going away! You can't shelter yourself or hide from it, or ignore it and hope it magically disappears. Those are fantasies. And if you let it start to consume and overtake you, then your brain and body will be wasting valuable energy. Wouldn't you rather that energy be devoted to something else, like, say, digestion and burning fat? The reality is that stress is here to stay, so you have to figure out how to conquer and convert it. Otherwise, you'll exist in a state of tension, dread, and paralysis-by-analysis. For me, vibrancy is really about stress management, so that our brain and bodies don't zap our chi!

My go-to stress reducers and keys to vibrancy? Communication, exercise, meditation, sleep, and sex!

COMMUNICATION: LET IT ALL HANG OUT

Why do it alone? And by "it," I mean life and all that it throws at you. It's healthy to communicate and express how you feel, and let yourself openly emote, to the people in your life who you trust and are close to. Your friends and family can listen, commiserate, and offer you valuable perspective on what you're going through. I can't get through life without talking it out, working it out, or crying it out. At times, I can feel like I'm oversharing, but holding it in just leaves me replaying the stress, pain, or situation over and over again. Did you know a burst of emotion lasts only ninety seconds? If you're repeatedly feeling an emotion until you're in "emo mode," you're going to find yourself in a self-destructive loop. Bottling it up is dangerous, too. When have you done that and not eventually exploded? And of course, you might turn to unhealthy food to comfort and console yourself. Food may provide a temporary escape or reprieve, but trust me, you can't eat your way out of stress! So find a person—a friend, sibling, parent, therapist, or partner—who you can talk to about what's stressing you out and who can help you work through your emotions.

EXERCISE:
HOW MOVEMENT SUSTAINS YOU

I know, you really don't need (or want) another person to tell you that exercise is good for you, right? I know you know! But it's worth repeating. Sweating equals less stress, and exercise boosts your metabolism, helps you lose weight, and keeps your body and brain healthy. I'll acquaint you with some basic science behind exercise, which I think will help motivate you to add some physical activity into your life. You don't have to train for an Ironman triathlon, go heavy into CrossFit, or put yourself through grueling seven-day-a-week workouts. But consistently incorporating some form of exercise as part of your Fab Four lifestyle will pay huge dividends, both physically and in terms of reducing your overall stress levels.

In its most basic form, exercise can either be aerobic or anaerobic, and we need both for optimal fitness. Aerobic exercise gets your heart pumping and the oxygen flowing through your cardiovascular system (your lungs, heart, and blood)—think cardio. Any form of exercise that raises your heart rate for an extended period of time is considered to be aerobic: distance walking, jogging or running, swimming, cycling/spin, rowing, sustained time on the elliptical machine, cross-country skiing, Vinyasa yoga, and even tai chi. Aerobic exercises tend to emphasize endurance and stamina, and are usually considered less "intense" than anaerobic exercise. Aerobic exercise strengthens your heart and lungs, burns fat, and reduces your risk of diabetes.

Aerobic exercise uses oxygen to fuel the exertion. Keep in mind that getting into fat-burning range isn't as easy as running out your front door. Most people run too hard (and run out of oxygen) or fuel incorrectly. If you are a runner, consider working with a lab to get your exact aerobic range, and use a heart rate monitor to help you stay in range. If you are just looking to add a little cardio to help burn fat, the best time to do it aerobically is first thing in the morning on an empty stomach or after a twenty-minute weight-training workout.

Anaerobic exercises are short, intense bursts of activity in which your oxygen levels aren't sufficient to help fuel the exertion. Exercises that use your muscles at a high intensity for a *short period* of time are considered anaerobic: weightlifting, kettlebells, resistance training, jumping rope, sprinting, downhill skiing, or one to three minutes of boxing/kickboxing. With intense exertion, there is a limited amount of oxygen available; the body must then turn to muscles for their stored glycogen. Because anaerobic workouts target muscle growth, they're the best choice if your fitness goals center on strength, muscle mass, or overall protection of your skeleton and bones.

A lot of my female clients are reluctant to do any weightlifting or kettlebell exercises for fear of bulking up or gaining weight. But listen to me, ladies—lifting weights (or using your body weight for resistance) consistently will always help you lean, lengthen, and tighten. In addition, **muscle strength stokes your metabolism**—a pound of muscle burns 50 to 75 calories daily, whereas a pound of fat burns only up to 5. Gaining strength will give you the most food freedom! Adding an anaerobic kettlebell routine might mean you weigh a pound more, but just watch your jean size go down. If you aren't hitting goals, focus on strength in the gym, or squats, lunges, and planks at home to help build your muscle mass. My trainer Mike Alexander of Madfit says, "Most bulk is not muscle, it's fat. If you can pinch it, you can lose it." You will not bulk!

Despite the distinction between aerobic and anaerobic exercise, almost all activities and sports actually use both systems. Think of your muscles as your gas tanks. When you exercise, you draw from your tanks and use glycogen as energy. When your tanks are empty, your body will burn fat as fuel. But if you can't access fat storage fast enough, it's a slower process and can cause you to hit the wall. Furthermore, you won't burn fat if you are using sugary drinks, gels, and bars because your body will prioritize that easily available fuel, and in addition, the presence of insulin will prevent lipolysis (fat breakdown). If you are an athlete or marathoner, I recommend UCAN SuperStarch products, which slowly release fuel, keep blood glucose balanced, and prevent high blood sugar spikes and excess insulin.

A good example of exercises that combine aerobic and anaerobic benefits are high-intensity interval training (HIIT), activities such as Spin or CrossFit, and yoga classes that include weights. These types of exercises include sustained cardio movement, as well as bursts of strengthening with weights. The same goes for sports like soccer, tennis, basketball, and football: sprinting, dodging, and jumping, as well as longer periods of sustained running or movement that combine both anaerobic and aerobic conditioning.

Such combo exercises such as HIIT have an added bonus. Because anaerobic activities produce excess post-exercise oxygen consumption, or EPOC (informally called afterburn), they keep your body burning calories after you've finished your workout. EPOC occurs so that your body can replenish its oxygen supply. It's as if your body is going for a light jog (even though you aren't) after lifting.

The bottom line? Choose exercises that challenge your muscles while also getting your heart pumping and strengthening your endurance and stamina. Thankfully, the majority of classes and workouts today incorporate both aerobic and anaerobic exercise and can be done at any time of the day. Together, this combo will keep you toned, energetic, and insulin sensitive. Cardio activities will not only keep your heart healthy but also burn fat. Balancing cardio with strength training and high-intensity activities will help you build tone, strength, and metabolism.

MOVEMENT TO SHIFT YOUR MIND-SET

One of the fastest ways to change your mental state is through movement. Tony Robbins is known for explaining how using your physiology can bio-chemically change how you feel: **"Emotion is created by motion."** Basically, we can use movement to actually change our mental and emotional state. Starting your day with a walk, jog, yoga class, or another form of light aerobic exercise allows you to not only physically move but also emotionally move the negative, unaligned thoughts from your mind. (Plus, getting out the door and moving before breakfast gives you the tank-dumping, muscle-strengthening, and insulin-sensitivity benefits mentioned above.) It works any time of day.

My go-to for de-stressing and shifting out of a mental or emotional funk zone is an afternoon or evening yoga class. I like Vinyasa flow classes with upbeat music that makes me want to sing. Not only does yoga reduce training-induced stress, but it increases flexibility, muscle strength, and muscle tone, all while improving respiration, energy, and vitality. Try it—you might love it! In my experience, yoga and Spin instructors get you moving, infuse you with positivity, and give you that spark of inspiration to conquer life's challenges.

WHAT DO YOU LIKE TO DO?

We all have different exercise preferences. My advice is to move and work out the way *you* like to, whether it's lifting at a gym, twerking it out in a dance class, or jogging around the neighborhood. And don't be afraid to try something new. You'll be surprised by the different muscle groups you work when you try something like Pilates, yoga, or resistance training. The key is to be *consistent*. I change up what I do all the time, but I get moving at least five days a week. Honestly, that's the most consistent part of my exercise routine!

One way to encourage your consistency is to pay in advance! Workout apps, online guides, and membership-based workout classes that make you sign up and pay ahead of time are great tools for motivation. But in order to really get in the habit of regular workouts, you've got to enjoy what you are doing and/or those you're doing it with. That's why I gravitate to yoga and Spin—the music is good, I feed off the other class members' energy, and I find the instructors give some of the best, soulful life advice. Nowadays we have so many options. You're bound to find at least a couple of activities that are fun and motivate you. Making it fun means making it consistent.

What do you enjoy? Walking, jogging, running, hiking, HIIT, yoga, cycling, Spin, swimming, home workouts, Pilates, CrossFit, weightlifting, kettlebells, dance, Bar Method classes, kickboxing, or sports like soccer, tennis, or basketball. Cue into the kinds of exercise you actually enjoy and then do some research on what kinds of classes, sports, or workouts offer that same kind of enjoyment. If you live in a city that has ClassPass, it might be a great way to find something new. You pay one monthly fee and get to try new gyms and different classes. I've done this a few times when I get bored or plateau (everyone plateaus, by the way!), or if I'm going to be staying in another city for a week.

Here's a quick quiz to help you figure out what you like . . . and what you don't. Use your responses to follow the dots!

1. Do you like to spend time outdoors?
2. Do you like participating in team sports?
3. Does working out with others motivate or discourage you?
4. Would you rather work out less than 30 minutes more often or less often?

GREAT POST-WORKOUT BRIDGE SNACKS

One of the benefits of HIIT and weightlifting is how they stoke your metabolism (EPOC!) and help you burn fat and use excess sugar that's floating around in your blood. You're also storing some of this excess sugar as glycogen in your muscles. So when you work out, you bring down your blood sugar. But working out hard means you sometimes need a post-workout bridge snack to get to the next meal, or as a way to help add muscle mass. Although I generally dissuade my clients from snacking, if you aren't going to eat a real meal within 90 to 120 minutes, or are looking to build strength, I recommend these delicious and protein-rich snacks:

- Half-size Fab Four Smoothie (like a "Roadie," page 200) with 10 to 15g of protein.
- Chocolate chia seed pudding. If you're looking for something a little more solid, try this recipe. It's one of my clients' favorite snacks, unbelievably easy to make ahead, and includes the benefits of the Roadie.
    1. Mix 1 scoop of chocolate protein powder with 1 cup unsweetened almond milk.
    2. Add 1 tablespoon MCT oil or coconut oil and 1 tablespoon chia seeds.
    3. Shake it up, then refrigerate. After about an hour, it should have a pudding consistency. Enjoy!
- Salmon salad (page 121) on cucumber slices. This snack will boost your body's omegas, satisfy your belly (and your bloodstream), and restore your energy after a serious workout.
- Apples (celery or berries) and nut butter. I like saving my fruit consumption of the day for my daily smoothie or dessert, or after I work out. Apples and almond butter are one of my go-tos after weights, HIIT, or anaerobic workout classes. This delicious snack serves up a dose of protein and fat on a carbohydrate- and fiber-dense apple slice. You're getting macronutrients and sweet, salty, and crunchy goodness all in one bite.
- Half an avocado, stuffed. One of my new faves! Here are some tantalizing combinations to try on top of half an avocado: 1 scoop of egg, tuna, or salmon salad; 2 tablespoons of your favorite hummus; 1 baked egg.

5. When you were in the playground as a child, where were you most likely to be found: the swings, playing tag, hopscotch, the rings, climbing . . . ?

6. Do you like to sweat?

7. Do you like to exert yourself and feel your heart pumping?

8. Do you like to move slowly with long stretches?

9. Do you like to beat your last performance?

10. Do you like to spend time alone?

11. Do you like to walk and talk at the same time?

12. Do you like to shop by yourself or with a friend?

13. Do you like to follow someone or make up your own routine?

14. Do you prefer having long, slender muscles or a strong, sturdy body?

15. Do you like to try new things or do you have tried-and-trues you love?

MEDITATION

Meditation isn't just for monks—it's for everyone! There are a ton of different ways to try it. You can do it on your own with an app or online course, join a group or go to a studio, or even find a teacher to work with you one-on-one. Whatever works best for you, your style, and your schedule. And meditation isn't just some fad or hippie-dippie fluff. There's very real science that has demonstrated its amazing health benefits.

Recent studies suggest that meditation both decreases cortisol levels (the "stress" hormone) and improves your overall stress response. It can also increase the levels of some of our most important neurotransmitters: dopamine and serotonin, the "reward" and "happy" hormones that elevate our moods and literally make us feel happier (sans cupcake!); and acetylcholine, which is a memory-and-learning booster.

Meditation calms the nervous system without triggering your adrenals. The effect is heightened awareness, a sense of well-being, and a boost in memory and learning. Meditation has also been shown to have other tangible health benefits, such as improved immunity, lower inflammation, and decreased pain. Further, brain-imaging studies show meditation increases gray matter in the brain, sharpens attention, and improves memory.

Transcendental meditation (chanting), Zen or seated meditation (with an instructor), or primordial sound meditation (vibrational sound) can make meditation seem intimidating, but there are some easier gateway types of mediation that can help you get into it. Like eating your Fab Four and working out, you don't need to be perfect or a professional—you just need to be consistent. Try the two methods below to see which one piques your interest. Need to be held accountable? Download an app like Calm, Omvana, Headspace, or OMG I Can Meditate to stay consistent.

Mindfulness Meditation

This classic style of meditation is the "gateway" to all the other forms. It's great for beginners and can be done anywhere. The intention is to bring focus to and release tension in the physical body through your breathing.

First, close your eyes and bring your attention to the inhalation and exhalation of air. Focus on each breath. Then start a body scan. As you continue to breathe, focus your attention on your toes and slowly work your way up your body, thinking about each part with heightened awareness. Release tension on exhales and send love on inhales. Give each body part 30 to 60 seconds of attention. Get comfortable and sink into the moment. You can do this seated or lying down and be done in 2 to 3 minutes.

♦

Focused Meditation

Focused meditation can be described as an "attention meditation technique," where we choose to focus on one thing to the exclusion of all else. The singular focus allows us to quiet our busy minds and feel peace. The object can be a person, place, thing, idea, or mantra. This is my go-to meditation, and I normally throw the sound of ocean waves on my headphones and "find my beach" (without the Corona). The goal isn't to fight your thoughts, it's to just refocus when you drift back to your to-do list.

YOUR MIND IS A POWERFUL THING

Mindfulness is a state of being that requires constant practice. Here are two other things that help me de-stress and stay connected to myself in a soulful way. You might enjoy them, too!

1. JOURNALING

Most mornings, I try to start my day by journaling. I learned this technique from the now-classic *The Artist's Way* by Julia Cameron; she calls them morning pages. Cameron describes the process like this: "These are three pages of longhand, stream-of-consciousness writing, done first thing in the morning. They are about anything and everything that crosses your mind and they are for your eyes only. Morning pages provoke, clarify, comfort and prioritize, which helps to synchronize the day at hand." Give it a try!

2. RECONNECTING TO ONE OF YOUR SMART GOALS

Remind yourself of your SMART goals (see page 78) and choose one to drill down on. When I work one on one with clients, we dig in and clarify what needs to be done next—whether it's improved sleep, drinking more water, working out, meditating, calling a friend, or making the next meal a healthy one. We often set too many vague or unattainable goals that end in failure and create a cloud of stress and anxiety. Making and reviewing SMART goals is a stress-busting habit that will help you convert goals into realistic, actionable daily tasks. You'll make good habits easily, without overwhelming yourself with the big picture.

3. BREATHING

I mean it! Sometimes, in the constant rush of our days, we forget to take big, deep breaths. At a stoplight? Breathe. At your desk? Breathe. After your first sip of morning coffee? Breathe. Flood your system with oxygen and let it be. Take one now. So good, right?

GET THYSELF TO SLEEP!

Sleep is a superpower. It's proven to reduce the risk of many chronic diseases, protect against illness, improve memory and mood, increase cognitive function, restore energy to the body and brain, and reduce stress levels. It helps keep us slim, too! Ever feel just a little "tighter" after a good night's rest? Well, as you may recall from chapter 4, we burn fat and lose weight when we sleep. Sleep plays a crucial role in maintaining proper metabolism, as well as blood sugar and hormone balance. If you're eating balanced Fab Four meals during the day, you're setting yourself up to lose weight at night, but if your sleep cycle is disrupted, this weight-losing boost might not happen.

So how can we improve our sleep and get more of that waist-slimming shut-eye? Well, it's not just about how much sleep we get. It turns out that when we go to bed, when we wake up, and the amount of light we're exposed to before bedtime all play significant roles as well.

A lot of what our body "does" is in response to the lightness or darkness of our environment. **Circadian rhythms** are biological processes that follow a roughly twenty-four-hour cycle, and the main external cue for these processes is the light-dark cycle of a day. Our bodies are regulated in response to the light and dark cycle. Our brain functioning, cellular functioning, hormonal cycles, and other processes all are impacted by circadian rhythms. If we disrupt the cycle, we disrupt our circadian rhythms. Unfortunately, we do this all the time! Simply put, it's too light at night. Artificial light allows us to stay awake long after sundown, and the blue light from televisions, computers, tablets, cell phones, and other screens only keeps us up and stimulated longer. All that blue light interferes with our sleep by suppressing melatonin production.

Melatonin is the hormone that makes you sleepy and keeps your circadian rhythm matched to the light-dark cycle. When it's dark, your body produces melatonin. When it's light, this production drops. Normally, melatonin levels begin to rise in the evening and remain high for most of the night. Then, in the early morning hours, those levels drop and the hormone cortisol is released, waking you up. You want a strong cortisol awakening response (CAR), which is about a 50 percent increase in your blood cortisol levels 30 to 60 minutes after you wake up in response to light.

As we age, our nighttime melatonin production can experience a natural decrease. However, blue light from artificial lighting and electronic devices actively *suppresses* melatonin production. If you're out late, up watching TV, or lying in bed on Instagram or Facebook, your body doesn't produce its normal levels of melatonin. When you finally turn off the lights, you may not fall asleep right away. Here's the kicker—if you have a circadian mismatch, you can actually *gain weight,* even with a better diet or more consistent workouts. Studies also show if you're trying to lose weight but living off rhythm, you may lose more muscle than fat mass, crave carbohydrates, and feel foggy-brained or irritated.

Melatonin-rich and on-rhythm sleep is the best cleanse your body will ever have—period! Sleep allows for DNA repair, decreases inflammation, and increases insulin sensitivity in muscles. When you wake up, your metabolism will be primed and ready to eat. Melatonin is also a potent antioxidant and DNA protector, and it helps regulate other hormones. In addition, without proper melatonin levels, oxidative stress goes haywire and you age faster. As the day goes on, we are less able to deal with oxidative stress and our body stores sugar in fat cells more easily.

So how do you make sure you get a good night's sleep and rediscover your circadian rhythm? You create a routine and try some of these easy tips.

> TIP: Have your one serving of fruit in the morning and quinoa in your mixed green salad at lunch.

1. **HUMAN BEDTIME.** Go to bed around the same time each night! This is part of the consistency you are going for. Of course, there will be late nights, but if you keep to your regular schedule on most nights, a slight deviation will not disrupt your sleep cycle.

2. **TECHNOLOGY BEDTIME.** Lower the lights and put away/turn off the technology at least two hours before bed, or at least wear anti–blue light glasses (see tip 6) and use the new "night shift" settings on computers, phones, and tablets. Artificial lights and the "off-gases" from electronic devices (no matter how small!) can disrupt our natural body clocks. It's not news that our brains and bodies are hardwired to sleep and rise in circadian rhythm. When the sun sets and the natural light fades, we naturally begin to shut down for the day. So, as part of your bedtime routine, lower the lights in your bedroom. If you're reading as a way to relax, use a soft reading lamp.

3. **BEDTIME ROUTINE.** If it works for toddlers, it can work for you, too! To wind down and relax, create a bedtime routine that starts one to two hours before you actually get under the sheets. Consider a bath or shower, listening to soft music (unless your spouse will sing to you), or reading a real book. Establishing a routine provides consistency and sets up a pattern that your brain and body will fall into.

4. **LIMIT MEALS BEFORE BEDTIME.** It's a good idea to stop eating or drinking at least three hours before going to bed, to give your body time to begin digestion and settle down for the night. Also, reducing carbohydrates at dinner can help minimize evening blood sugar and the proclivity for fat storage. This goes along with circadian nutrient timing. According to one study, a low-carbohydrate, protein-rich dinner best preserves lean tissue during weight loss.

5. **CONSIDER TAKING MELATONIN.** If you're really having trouble falling or staying asleep, many functional medicine practitioners suggest taking melatonin. This hormone is produced by our bodies in higher quantities up to around age ten or eleven, then we experience a decrease, even though we still need it in sufficient amounts to keep our circadian cycle working well. Consult your doctor. Starting with 1 to 3 milligrams approximately thirty minutes before going to bed might help your sleep.

6. **WEAR ANTI-BLUE LIGHT GLASSES.** New lenses that block blue light are proven to be very effective! They typically have an orange or amber tint. This is a huge advantage for working late, watching TV, or taking your phone to bed. The lenses should be worn after dark until you go to bed. Okay, so they may not look sexy, but the ends justify the means, right?

7. **AIM FOR EIGHT HOURS.** Aim for eight hours of sleep per night, but try your best to wake and go to bed with the sun. The closer you can get your sleep hours aligned with natural light-dark cycle of a day, the more benefits you'll reap.

8. **WAKE UP EARLY.** Wake up and go out into the sun to help reset your circadian rhythm. If you are planning to work out, try to do it outside.

9. **START THE DAY.** Don't delay! If you are off to work, drink your Fab Four Smoothie first thing in the morning with your car window or sunroof open so the sun can shine through on you. No sun? Consider purchasing a sunlight lamp for your office desk to get you back in the groove.

STAYING SEXUALLY HEALTHY

Sex may be part of a natural drive for reproduction, but it also plays an important role in stoking our vitality. I call it staying sexually healthy because it's so important for your overall wellness. Responsible and healthy sexual activity (whether you are with a partner or not) is a way to keep yourself open to pleasure, enjoyment, and the feel-good hormones your body naturally produces. It's also a key to vibrancy—a way to feel, look, and stay young and healthy, both inside and out. Remember the friend who walks into the party who emanates an inner glow? The other energy she's emitting is sexual confidence and the spark of a healthy sexual drive.

I'm no sexologist or sex therapist, but I think it's pretty obvious that not shying away from sex is just plain good for you! It can also have physical and emotional benefits, such as relieving stress, improving mood and sleep, improving cardiovascular health, strengthening the pelvic floor muscles, helping prevent cervical and urinary tract infections, and strengthening relationships. Further, staying aware of your sexual hormonal health—regardless of your age or situation—is key to experiencing a better overall quality of life.

Over time, work stress, emotional stress, lack of sleep, poor diet, and inadequate exercise can throw your hormones out of whack, ultimately leaving you with a low sex drive. In addition, food sensitivities, environmental toxins, and certain prescription drugs can rev up the production of cortisol (the "stress" hormone), which results in yet another blow to your libido. Fortunately, there's hope for turning things around and getting your hormones—and your love life—back on track, with no drugs required.

Let's take a closer look at how stress can impact our sex life. When we're stressed, our body produces cortisol. Cortisol is made in our adrenal glands by another hormone, called pregnenolone. Pregnenolone is the grandmother of all hormones—it's involved in creating many others, including our "sex" hormones (estrogen, testosterone, progesterone). The problem is, when we're under a great deal of stress, our adrenal glands are hyperstimulated and pregnenolone is so busy producing cortisol that the production of our sex hormones slows way down. The result is adrenal fatigue, which can lead to menstrual cycle issues, mood imbalances, and even infertility.

If your libido-boosting sex hormones need recharging, your doctor may try jump-starting your system with a prescription version of pregnenolone. This is known as the **replacement model** of rebalancing hormones—doctors will measure what's low and prescribe hormones to try to replace it. However, taking prescription hormones could potentially cause your body to stop producing those hormones naturally.

The other approach to rebalancing hormones, known as the **functional model,** determines the underlying cause of the problem and addresses it so that your hormones naturally rebalance without replacements. The functional model focuses on minimizing external and internal stressors and eating natural foods that support the production of sex hormones. Before treating a hormonal imbalance, check with your doctor to make sure there are no underlying conditions causing or contributing to the problem. Here are some functional-based tips to try.

To Combat External Stressors

- Sleep! Sleep allows our hormones to balance naturally and can increase your libido. Aim for eight hours per night in a cool, blacked-out room.
- If your responsibilities at work are causing high levels of stress, schedule a time with your boss to discuss your goals for the future and anything in your role that is especially stressful. Don't be afraid to ask. These days many companies are open to change and willing to put processes into place to

make their employees happy. A happier, less-stressed you is a more productive, efficient you. Your boss should want that!

- Steer your activities with friends in a healthy direction—choose hikes over happy hours.

- Acknowledge and invest in the relationships in your life that push you, support you, and hold you accountable to be your best self.

- Get moving! Take a long walk, go to a morning yoga class or Pilates, or sneak in a twenty-minute workout at lunch. All these exercises involve enough movement to help you stay lean and sweat (great for detoxing), but not so much that you're overworking your muscles and creating a surge in cortisol from training stress. If you like to work out hard, make sure you're getting adequate rest between sessions so training stress doesn't become chronic. Yes, more advice to sleep!

To Combat Internal Stressors

It's not just external stressors (such as an overflowing e-mail inbox) that trigger cortisol. Internal stressors such as food sensitivities, inflammation, and prescription drugs may also be contributing to your lack of libido.

- If you have food allergies, your body may be experiencing internal inflammation. Inflammation can increase cortisol production and thus affect your body's production of sex hormones. Take a food allergy test and see how you might need to change your diet.

- Try to limit the use of prescription drugs that kill gut bacteria and instead supplement with a quality probiotic supplement to increase your immune system and promote healthy bacteria, keeping inflammation to a minimum.

- Fatty acids like omega-3s to the rescue! By eating higher amounts of

omega-3, we can decrease cellular inflammation (thereby decreasing cortisol) and also increase our hormone receptor function, which helps control
and balance hormone levels.

• Cholesterol (in moderation) helps support pregnenolone production.
Foods such as egg yolks, cold-water fish (salmon, sardines, cod, herring),
and shellfish (shrimp, lobster, clams, calamari, oysters, mussels) offer a
healthy dose of cholesterol that will help to balance your hormones in a way
that won't overload your system the way prescription hormones might.

Responsible and healthy sexual activity has important emotional and physical benefits. Sex is a natural endorphin releaser and de-stresser. So many of us
might put off sex, thinking that we are too tired, we'll get to it next week, or that,
since we don't have a partner, it's not worth the bother. Ladies—stop right there!
Your sexual vibe is a strong conduit to your vibrancy.

10
BADASS BEAUTY— INSIDE AND OUT

BEAUTY IS MORE THAN skin deep. It emerges from all that is within us— how we think, how we feel, and how we nourish ourselves. It's a product of all of us, and it starts from the inside. Our outer beauty will shine only if we replenish, restore, and augment our inner beauty. That means taking good care of what's happening on the inside of our bodies, because in turn the inside will take care of the outside. Indeed, our skin (the largest organ of our body) is a vivid, living reflection of how we're treating ourselves. In this chapter, you're going to learn how to nourish your body from the inside out so that your skin, hair, and overall aura reflect good, clean health. It's a continuation of the inner equilibrium you've been striving for with your Fab Four Smoothie and Fab Four meals, as well as the lifestyle, vibrancy, and other tools that complete the Fab Four lifestyle. All these tips apply to men as well as women. You guys might not think of yourself as "beautiful," but handsome is as handsome does!

YOUR GUT HEALTH

Outer beauty starts in your gut. Yep, your gut! The health of your gut significantly influences the health and glow of your skin. The answer for clear skin is a dirty gut. And by dirty, I mean full of "good" or "healthy" gut bacteria.

Our bodies are full of microorganisms. Full! In fact, there are more than ten times more microbial cells than human cells in our bodies, weighing in at a total of approximately twenty pounds. This ecological community inside us is known as the **human microbiome**, and it's closely connected to our health and wellness. Some of these microorganisms do us good (so-called good or healthy gut bacteria), while others do us harm (such as candida and yeast). In 2008, the National Institutes of Health (NIH) created the Human Microbiome Project to identify and characterize the various microorganisms found in humans. By studying these microbial communities, researchers hoped to gain a better understanding of the role they play in human health and disease. One of the five body sites emphasized by the Human Microbiome Project was the gut.

Our "good" or "healthy" gut bacteria do all sorts of helpful things for our digestion, health, and overall wellness. As such, the gut is an ecosystem we must nourish, support, and feed to keep healthy. Unfortunately, antibiotics, poor eating habits, and even birth control pills have negatively affected the delicate balance of this ecosystem. These inputs can increase yeast and candida (not good!), and induce the release of the peptide Substance P, which plays a major role in various skin conditions. Dysbiosis, or microbial imbalance, has also been shown in 61 percent of acne sufferers.

The healthiest way to nourish healthy gut bacteria is to keep them fed! Those healthy bacteria will protect you from the outside world, stubborn "bad" bacteria that can invade your system, and the side effects of medicines.

Your good gut bacteria eat resistant starches (aka prebiotics), which can be found in vegetables (squash, yam, asparagus, sunchoke), legumes (beans, lentils, peas), and seeds (chia, flax). The Fab Four help you get enough of these "gut-builders" through the greens and fiber portions of your plate. There are four types of resistant starches, and multiple types can be found in the same foods:

- Type 1 has a cell wall that resists digestion.
- Type 2 is found in raw or unripe starchy foods.
- Type 3 is formed through retro-gradation, or a process of cooking and cooling starch.
- Type 4 is chemically man-made (not recommended).

Feeding prebiotics to your good bacteria daily helps ensure you have healthy digestion, immune system function, and bowel movements. It will also help reduce the ability of disease-causing microorganisms (such as candida or yeast) to populate the colon. Most important, the digestion of resistant starch by our healthy bacteria provides fuel for our cells, including gases and short-chain fatty acids like butyrate, which is anti-inflammatory (it decreases cell permeability) and anticancer, and supports your metabolism. By incorporating unmodified resistant starch, you may lower blood sugar, make your insulin more sensitive, and better your chances to lose weight.

You can supplement prebiotics naturally, without pills. This beneficial fiber exists out there in nature; you just need to eat it or drink it in a Be Well Smoothie. In your smoothie, you can add up to 1 teaspoon per day of resistant starch (see page 139), such as unmodified potato starch or plantain or green banana flour. Other ways to make sure you get enough of these naturally occurring prebiotics is to include leafy greens (which contain a sugar that literally feeds good bacteria!), raw asparagus or dandelion greens, sunchokes, cauliflower, raw garlic, raw leeks, and cooked or raw onions.

Just remember, too much of a good thing can also be bad. Overfeeding bacteria can cause gut discomfort, gas, and cramping. Avoid prebiotics (or consult your doctor) if you suffer from SIBO or have been instructed to follow a FODMAPS diet. Moderation and consistency are key!

Prebiotics are not to be confused with *probiotics*. Probiotics are live bacteria that support your gut health and wellness. They're more of the good stuff—and it's the good bacteria in our gut that is the touchpoint between our epigenetics and genetics. Our healthy gut bacteria keeps us well by:

- synthesizing folate (rate limiting factor in methylation) and vitamin K
- improving mineral absorption from food
- producing Short-Chain Fatty Acids (SCFA's—like butyrate) which enforce the gut barrier and mediate local and systemic inflammation
- improving transit time of feces through the colon; positive influence on transit of luminal contents by peristalsis
- competing with pathogenic microbes for nutrients and binding sites on mucosal epithelial cells
- modulating our immune response
- producing our key neurotransmitters
- reducing acne and skin related disorders

There are a few different ways to incorporate them into your diet. One way is in pill form with a probiotic supplement. Here are a few tips for selecting the right one for you:

ENSURE YOUR PROBIOTIC CONTAINS HUMAN-DERIVED STRAINS. You'd be surprised to learn that strains come from all places; soil, pigs, and even dolphins. Many of the "soil-based organisms" were actually first developed for use in fish feed, veterinary practices, and the livestock industry with little to no testing on a human microbiome.

ENSURE PROVEN SURVIVAL THROUGH DIGESTION THAT ENDS IN THE COLON. Probiotics are measured in Colony-Forming Units (CFU's). Companies either list survival on their label at time of manufacture, or sometimes at time of purchase but true survival should be measured by the quantity that make it to the microbiome.

LOOK FOR STRAIN-SPECIFIC CFU COUNT. Many labels will list the overall quantity of probiotics (i.e. 20 billion CFU) without the quantity of each individual strain. Unfortunately, this is a labeling loophole, as the blend could be 99% Lactobacillus Acidophilus (one of the cheapest strains to manufacture) with only trace quantities of the other strains.

MORE CFU DOESN'T MEAN BETTER. Probiotics die off during digestion on the logarithmic scale instead of linear scale (i.e., 10^3 or 3 log die off) which is actually 1000x. So the difference between 100 billion CFU and 10 billion CFU (1 log) isn't more significant than the die off rate (which could easily result in 1000x to 10,000x die off).

REFRIGERATED PROBIOTICS AREN'T BETTER. Refrigeration means the company couldn't figure out how to stabilize their microbes and are passing the burden onto the consumer. Unfortunately, this means your probiotics could be breaking down during transport to the store, home, or while traveling.

Looking for my recommendation on what probiotic to take? Seed is the first company to verify the survival of their product (with their stabilization and delivery system) through 5 stages of gastrointestinal transit ending in the gut microbiota. The algae-based delivery system allows their probiotics to survive digestion and also stabilizes them up to 40 degrees Celsius (104 Fahrenheit).

Another way to incorporate probiotics is to eat fermented foods. Although we don't know for sure if these foods are delivering any "live" probiotics to the intestines fermentation makes our food more nutritious and easier to digest.

You probably won't be surprised that my favorite fermented foods are fiber-rich vegetables like sauerkraut and kimchi (fermented cabbage). Add to your diet fermented drinks like coconut kefir and yogurt (fermented coconut milk) and kombucha (plain fermented tea) occasionally. Many commercially fermented drinks are loaded with sugar that can interfere with blood sugar balance, so enjoy them with a complete Fab Four meal. Although the fermentation process breaks down the lactose in dairy (lowering the carbohydrate and sugar content, and helping decrease the allergen lactose), I still opt for my fiber-rich fermented foods first. Vegetable fermentation breaks down the food, making nutrients and minerals more bioavailable in the body.

THE CLEANSING TOOLBOX

One of the biggest health trends of the last decade has been the explosion of cleanses. Some have weird names (Ayurveda kitchari), some *seem* as if they must be good for you (only juice), and some seem a little insane (lemon water and cayenne pepper). There is no shortage of options out there, many of which promise instant weight loss and a complete detox for the body. Often, however, aggressive cleanses are not biologically sound and leave you full of insulin, protein deprived, and emotionally frazzled. For example, an all-juice cleanse is a weeklong roller coaster of blood sugar spikes and crashes.

In reality, our body is in a constant state of cleansing itself of the toxins and impurities we take in. And we take in a lot—from the food we ingest, our interactions with the environment, and products that contain chemicals. We have two major systems (elimination and excretion) and four major organs (lungs, skin, large intestine, and kidneys) that have significant detox functions.

- Our lungs rid the body of carbon dioxide through our breath, which you can augment with meditation, yoga, or breathing exercises.
- Our skin rids the body of excess water, heat, and salt, which you can boost with a workout or sauna session.
- Our large intestine rids the body of solid waste, including good and bad bacteria, which you can help along by sipping on calorie-dense, fiber-rich liquid meals like the Fab Four Smoothie, soups, and fat tea (tea blended with coconut oil or MCT oil, ghee, or grass-fed butter, like Irish Kerry Gold).
- Finally, our kidneys get rid of bacteria and other chemicals through urine, which you can support by staying hydrated and drinking plenty of water.

We are constantly detoxing, so to say you're "cleansing" is always true. We can help these systems get rid of waste and potentially harmful toxin buildup by supporting these organs naturally. A few small changes can go a long way toward helping your body do its daily job. So stop swinging from binge to cleanse and instead use this cleansing toolbox to autocorrect back into balance after a late night, a wine-country weekend, a cross-country trip, or a stressful work week.

1. **SLEEP, SLEEP, SLEEP.** (If you've forgotten already, check out page 217!)
2. **HYDRATE.** Drinking water slowly throughout the entire day will allow your body to use nature's elixir effectively for detoxification, weight loss, fatigue relief, headache prevention, and better skin health—all without diluting digestion. Aim for half your body weight in ounces, drinking 12 to 24 ounces before breakfast and between lunch and dinner, and sip only what you need

during your actual meals. Many factors affect hydration, so if you work out, drink lots of caffeine, or plan to spend your day in the sun, up your intake. Inadequate hydration has been linked with elevated body mass index (BMI) and obesity. Here are two quick water-related tips:

- Keep a chlorophyll dropper in your purse to make green water! If you recall from your grade school science class, chlorophyll is the green pigment responsible for photosynthesis. Adding just a few drops to your water can help control hunger, cravings, and body odor (even that one we women don't talk about). It's also a super-potent antioxidant that promotes healing and cleansing, including binding to heavy metals and helping kill off candida.

- Add a squeeze of lemon to your water! When you're not sipping on green water, go ahead and ask for a small plate of sliced lemons. Although acidic in nature, lemons are alkaline in your body. Warm lemon water first thing the morning hydrates your body naturally, and lemons purify the liver.

3. **DRINK A FRUIT-FREE KETO FAB FOUR SMOOTHIE (PAGE 142).** Start your day with a Fab Four Smoothie rich in MCT. Not only do medium-chain triglycerides help produce ketones and quick brain fuel, the lauric acid will kill candida and yeast overgrowth. Many people don't realize when they have a yeast overgrowth, and since it feeds on sugar, a big night out with wine or indulging a sweet tooth could promote its growth. To maintain gut balance, incorporate coconut oil (a source of MCT) into cooking and take a tablespoonful daily. And because the medium-chain triglycerides in coconut oil increase twenty-four-hour energy output (studies show by as much as 5 percent), you can lose even more weight while sleeping! That may not sound like much, but long term, it can be significant. This is why many of my clients make a habit of including at least 1 tablespoon of MCT-rich fat in their morning smoothie.

4. **BREAKFAST = BREAK THE FAST.** Let your body do its job at night! Eating dinner too late can cause leptin (the "satiety" hormone) to signal to the

brain that no energy is required, and thus no fat burning will occur until the early morning hours, if at all. Also, a big meal before bed can interfere with sleep, causing an imbalance of hunger hormones and overeating the following day. So between dinner and breakfast, try to get a complete twelve hours of fasting in. After all, to break a fast, you need to be fasting in the first place! If you eat dinner at seven P.M., try to make it to seven A.M., then jump-start your metabolism with a Fab Four Smoothie.

5. **MAKE SUPPER SUPPLEMENTAL.** Your body is less able to process foods for energy in the evening, when fat cells are more insulin-sensitive. This is why my plan encourages eating the majority of your carbohydrates earlier in the day and winding down in the evening. You will not miss food if you are *fed!* However, in order not to be hungry at night, you must stay in balance during the day. Here are a few dinner tools:

- **INTERMITTENT FASTING.** If you want to partake in this diet phenomenon, do it right: skip dinner intermittently. If you decide to pass on dinner once or twice a week, have a calorically dense, fructose-free, and fat-rich Fab Four Smoothie for breakfast.

- **FAT FAST.** Swap dinner for bone broth (chicken or beef), fat tea (page 231), or collagen- or gelatin-rich puree. All these fat-rich liquid meals can prevent aggressive cleansing side effects such as migraines, nausea, insomnia, and brain fog but offer the benefits of a liquid meal, light dinner, and balanced blood sugar. A liquid fast would be a coconut cream vegetable puree. There are companies that will send homemade bone broths to your door!

- **FAST FAST.** Complete a once-yearly four- to five-day fast. Dr. Longo of USC has done research that shows that this type of a fast causes stem cells to turn on, shrinks the liver, and kills off 40 percent of the immune cells. The subsequent "refeeding" then triggers a complete rebuilding. Talk about a real cleanse!

- **GO GREEN.** Meatless Monday shouldn't mean swapping your bison steak for a "spike" of quinoa, sweet potato teriyaki bowl, or cauliflower corn tacos—these are not protein replacements! Instead, swap your meat for a detox salad full of water-rich vegetables and medicinal herbs to help chelate your body of heavy metals, regenerate liver cells, and hydrate your body slowly. Or try a blanched vegetable soup with garlic, herbs, and bone broth. Lightly blanched vegetables will maintain vitamins, and when you chew them, you'll release enzymes and calm hunger hormones.

6. **SKIN SUPPORT.** The largest organ on your body can help you detox. Here are a few of my favorite tips to do so!

- **EXFOLIATE DAILY.** Use a bath mitt or dry brush to exfoliate your skin in the morning or the evening. A few minutes all over your body will remove dead skin cells and let your skin breathe. This can stimulate blood flow and lymphatic drainage and potentially reduce cellulite.

- **THERMOGENESIS.** Visit a hot infrared sauna for forty-five minutes or cold cryotherapy chamber for two minutes. Both challenge your metabolism to bring your core temperature back to equilibrium. A nice infrared in the evening is one of my favorite treats. You burn calories, sweat, speed up your metabolism, clear up your skin (including the appearance of cellulite), relieve joint and muscle aches and pain, boost your immune system, and remove toxins. I will go after a hard day when I don't have the energy I need to work out. Don't forget to bring a good book and some water in a non-BPA container! Cryotherapy involves exposing the body (as a whole or partially) to sub-zero conditions. It's known to boost cell life, decrease pain, lower inflammation, and improve your general health. It might be the longest two minutes of your life, but it's worth the chill.

◆

TAKING IT A STEP FURTHER: THE FAB FOUR CLEANSE

We all get run down, and when we do, our eating habits tend to slide. The result is feeling bloated or inflamed, seeing blemishes and breakouts on our skin, and having little or no energy. At these times it's natural to want to dedicate ourselves to a really healthy two- or three-day period to get back on track. My version of a cleanse is an autocorrect strategy that you can use all the time—and you'll still be able to eat! I do this on a regular basis, whenever I feel the need to make a rapid adjustment, such as after a wedding, a long weekend of fun, or a week of eighteen-hour workdays.

The Fab Four Cleanse helps you repopulate your colon with healthy bacteria, eliminate inflammation, stabilize blood sugar, and quickly shed unwanted weight. We remove inflammatory foods and add supplements needed for digestion, recovery, and metabolism. You need to stay balanced, sleep well, and keep your muscles, brain, and cells fed. Here's how I do it:

1. Eliminate the following foods (*denotes foods associated with food intolerance, autoimmune disease, and inflammation):
   - Gluten and grains*
   - Dairy*
   - Corn*
   - Soy*
   - Sugar/sugar alternatives*
   - Eggs*
   - Legumes (including peanuts)*
   - Coffee, soda, alcohol
   - Nightshades (tomatoes, eggplants, peppers, mushrooms)

- Fruit (If weight loss isn't a goal, you can incorporate ¼ cup organic berries daily.)

2. Supplement with the following:

- Probiotics: Take a probiotic daily.

- Enzymes: Digestive enzymes help your body break down your meals to release nutrients. This antiaging supplement is great for times of stress, travel, large meals, or cleansing. They are kept at room temperature and great to have on hand.

- Magnesium: For constipation.

- Vitamin D: If blood tests show low vitamin D, make sure to take a supplement.

In order to cleanse efficiently, you need to keep track of what you are consuming to make sure you are getting enough nutrition. Follow the breakdown below and copy and paste this as a guide into your Fab Four Notebook.

TIPS TO BEAUTIFY YOUR SKIN

The key to plump, smooth, and blemish-free skin comes down to taking care of it each and every day. The tips below are simple and will help you avoid breakouts, dry patches, and small lines around your eyes, forehead, or mouth. Make them a habit and you'll be amazed at how rejuvenated and revitalized your skin will be.

1. **CLEANSE YOUR SKIN.** Our outer skin is in a constant, active state of detox. When the outer skin becomes irritated, clogged, or congested, you will see the side effects on your skin (blemishes, rashes, and other delights). What you won't see is the inflammation inside your body, which is also a

CLEANSE DAY #_____ OF 21

Breakfast Smoothie // _____   Time _____

Components //

Protein _____

Greens _____

Water _____

Protein _____

Enzymes _____

_____

problem. These buildups will prematurely age the skin, causing wrinkles and sagging. You need to cleanse your skin twice daily with a pH-balanced, nonabrasive cleanser. Once a week you should gently exfoliate your skin to slough away dead skin and help it naturally restore itself.

2. **NOURISH YOUR SKIN.** The key to glowing skin is to understand the important role of our diet, including healthy fats. We cannot expect to

magically have plump, happy skin without addressing what we eat. Fat is essential for producing hormones, absorbing fat-soluble vitamins, hydrating skin from the inside out, and effectively balancing blood sugar. When our blood sugar is under control, we can help prevent hormonal breakouts caused by increased androgen levels. Healthy fats provide our body with the cholesterol and fatty acid precursors to balance hormones naturally. To help your body get what it needs, try incorporating these healthy fats into your daily routine:

- **AVOCADO.** Avocados contain monounsaturated fat that helps hydrate and shield the skin. In addition to acting as a natural moisturizer, avocados are associated with antiaging due to xanthophyll, an antioxidant and carotenoid with DNA damage protection. Avocados are also a primary source of vitamin E, which stimulates collagen production and benefits skin elasticity. They also help stabilize blood sugar, allowing your body to release fat, protect lean muscle, and increase energy. Avocado is a great add to any meal and even the perfect blood-sugar-stabilizing bridge snack as a dip with vegetables. Topically, avocado oil absorbs easily and can replace coconut oil as a lotion.

- **EGG YOLK.** One egg yolk contains thirteen essential nutrients, which makes it a superfood for your skin—on the inside and out! The yolk is rich in B vitamins, vitamins A and E, and selenium—all of which are important for vital cell function. Not only are egg yolks a fabulous source of protein, they are also a natural source of biotin, aka the "beauty vitamin" that promotes healthier skin, hair, and nails. Looking for a quick face mask? Simply fork-whisk an egg white until foamy, apply it to your freshly cleansed skin, and leave it to work for 2 to 15 minutes. Carefully take off the mixture with a warm washcloth when your skin begins to tingle or tighten.

- **COCONUT OIL.** Give your skin some love with a dollop of coconut oil! Bacteria begone! I even make a sugar-free freezer fudge out of it (see page 134)!

When ingested, coconut oil bypasses the liver and is used for energy instead of being converted into triglycerides. Further, the lauric acid (a potent anti-fungal) contained in coconut oil also helps to balance gut bacteria by killing off excess yeast and candida, which can contribute to breakouts. This luscious oil easily removes makeup, takes the place of body lotion, and can be mixed with equal parts cocoa butter for a quick DIY lip gloss.

- **GHEE OR PASTURE-RAISED BUTTER.** Full of CLA and butyric acid, ghee (clarified butter) and pasture-raised butter are processed by the liver and used for energy that can keep you satiated through the next meal. This healthy fat is also high in vitamin A, a natural skin clarifier, and vitamin D, a first line of defense against the sun's harmful UV rays. Incorporate ghee or grass-fed butter into your daily routine by adding a tablespoon to roasted vegetables, to the pan when you cook eggs, or into a bulletproof coffee.

- **OMEGA-3.** Recent studies suggest an omega-3 deficiency contributes to chronic acne. Adequate levels of this anti-inflammatory fatty acid will not only keep your skin clear but also increase cell hydration from the inside out. An unbalanced ratio of omega-3 to omega-6 can also result in skin conditions. Either way, up the omega-3! Wild salmon is one of the best food sources for omega-3 fatty acids and protein. This fish is also known for its vitamin D and selenium, a mineral that protects the skin from the sun's harmful UV rays. Sardines, oysters, and mackerel are also excellent sources of omega-3 fatty acids.

3. **MOISTURIZE YOUR SKIN.** My best-kept secret to getting that dewy look is oiling my skin both internally and externally. By doing this a few nights a week, you will keep hydrated and looking dewy. A thin veil of simple oils calms, hydrates, and helps heal the skin. For the glowiest look, choose a topical oil to swipe onto clean skin, exfoliate only a couple of nights a week, and choose a pH-balanced face wash. My favorite oils are calendula oil, marula oil, and squalene oil, but your oil doesn't need to be fancy. If you're

taking a long plane flight, fly with a clean face, swipe on a thin oil and lip balm, then spritz your face with a hydrator to stay hydrated and land fresh.

4. **PROTECT YOUR SKIN.** By keeping your body well hydrated and ingesting antioxidants, you boost your built-in protecting agents, helping to fight against the sun and other environmental pollutants. Specifically, vitamins B, C, and D, as well as selenium, help your body and therefore your skin fight against free radical damage and give your organs the support they need to get rid of toxins.

Here are some of my other go-to topical skin boosters:

- **TOPICAL VITAMIN C:** You might find it in a product or on its own.
- **HYALURONIC ACID:** This powerful moisture replenisher comes in a cream or cleanser. My skin has done a 180 since I've begun using hyaluronic acid as part of my cleansing routine.
- **PURE OIL:** Pure forms of oil are wonderful ways to restore moisture and vibrancy to your skin; try calendula oil, marula oil, and squalene oil, which are easy for your skin to absorb.
- **COENZYME Q10:** Another antioxidant that the body produces is coenzyme Q10, which stimulates cell growth. As with many natural-producing substances, we stop producing coenzyme Q10 later in life (exactly when varies from person to person). Give yourself a boost by taking a supplement.
- **ALPHA-LIPOIC ACID.** Another antioxidant with medicinal properties, when applied as a cream, it helps the skin restore itself from environmental damage, including sun damage from UVA and UVB rays.

FOODS TO BOOST ANTIOXIDANT POWER

If you're living a Fab Four lifestyle and eating clean, you'll get most of your vitamins, minerals, and other antioxidants from the food you ingest. But the foods on the Fab Four program also contain substances that boost collagen and elastin, proteins in skin that diminish when we age. Take a look at these skin-boosting foods:

- **SARDINES.** These canned goodies are the ocean's gift to your skin. Loaded with vitamin B12 for cell regeneration and selenium for protection from sun damage, these small bites are powerful antioxidants. And because they're packed with phosphorus, omega-3 fatty acids, protein, and vitamin D, they help hydrate and plump from the inside out. They're also a good source of calcium, niacin, copper, vitamin B2, and choline. Choline is a member of the B vitamin family and useful in the fatty portions of cell membrane's production. B vitamins are essential for healthy skin and also responsible for the production of energy, collagen, and elastin. You could say that a can of sardines a day will keep the plastic surgeon away.

- **OYSTERS.** Omega-3 fatty acids, vitamin C, and calcium are all wrapped up in these small shells. Recent studies suggest an omega-3 deficiency may contribute to chronic acne, and that one serving (eight oysters) will deliver your daily need of 1000 milligrams. A beauty bonus: Zinc in oysters also keeps your nails, hair, and eyes healthy.

- **KALE.** This anti-inflammatory veggie is chock-full of antioxidants, vitamins A and C, fiber, and calcium. What's more, the beta-carotene delivers a youthful glow and neutralizes free radicals. Chop up kale for a summer salad, sauté it in olive oil for a tasty side dish, or add a little to your morning Fab Four Smoothie.

- **SPINACH.** This leafy green is loaded with lutein, which will keep your eyes sparkling for the camera! Spinach is also a good source of omega-3s, potassium, calcium, iron, magnesium, and vitamins B, C, and E. Kale and spinach not your thing? All leafy greens contain folate, which is a powerful nutrient used in DNA repair.

- **WILD BLUEBERRIES.** Packed with antioxidants, wild blueberries are also a great source of vitamin A, known to normalize oil production. Throw some blueberries in your chia seed pudding for a protein-packed breakfast, or add them to a spinach salad for lunch if your breakfast was fruit-free. Wild blueberries will be darker and smaller than cultivated blueberries. You can find them frozen at Whole Foods or Trader Joe's.
- **PARSLEY.** Known for supporting liver and kidney functions, parsley acts as a metabolism booster while removing toxins. Add it to your daily Fab Four Smoothie or sprinkle the milder flat-leaf version on a salad.
- **CILANTRO.** Cilantro is rich in antioxidants that prevent damage from free radicals and help the body purge "heavy metals" consumed in non-organic foods. Grow your own easily at home and add it to rice, salads, salsas, and dips.

FINAL NOTE

Dear friends,

Yes—you all feel like new friends! I am thrilled that you accompanied me on this journey. I hope that all this advice makes sense, will stick with you, and will motivate you to find your own happy place of balance, energy, and good vibes. I also hope that you enjoyed learning some science!

Please know that you can reach out to me with questions and comments on my website—I love being in touch with my ever-burgeoning posse of like-minded peeps!

Be well. Be beautiful. Be you!

Love,
Kelly

REFERENCES

As I've mentioned, I'm a bit of a research geek. I love combing through studies, articles in science and nutrition journals, and the latest research being published. In this section, I've gathered the most important and relevant scientific articles and studies that support the information and advice in *Body Love*. I've organized them by topic for ease of access. Please feel free to take a peek or refer friends or physicians to this reference list!

BLOOD SUGAR

Parker B, et al. (2002 Mar). Effect of a high-protein, high-monounsaturated fat weight loss diet on glycemic control and lipid levels in type 2 diabetes. *Diabetes Care.* 25(3):425–30.

Vuksan V, et al. (2010 Apr). Reduction in postprandial glucose excursion and prolongation of satiety: possible explanation of the long-term effects of whole grain Salba (Salvia Hispanica L.). *Eur J Clin Nutr.* 64(4):436–38. doi: 10.1038/ejcn.2009.159. Epub 2010 Jan 20.

FASTER METABOLISM

Baum JI, Gray M, Binns A. (2015 Oct) Breakfasts higher in protein increase postprandial energy expenditure, increase fat oxidation, and reduce hunger in overweight children from 8 to 12 years of age. *J Nutr.* 145(10):2229–35. doi: 10.3945/jn.115.214551. Epub 2015 Aug 12.

Blom WA, et al. (2006 Feb) Effect of a high-protein breakfast on the postprandial ghrelin response. *Am J Clin Nutr.* 83(2):211–20.

Pesta DH, and VT Samuel. (2014) A high-protein diet for reducing body fat: mechanisms and possible caveats. *Nutr Metab* (Lond). 2014; 11: 53. Published online 2014 Nov 19. doi: 10.1186/1743-7075-11-53. PMCID: PMC4258944.

Dulloo AG, Fathi M, Mensi N, Girardier L. (1996 Mar) Twenty-four-hour energy expenditure and urinary catecholamines of humans consuming low-to-moderate amounts of medium-chain triglycerides: a dose-response study in a human respiratory chamber. *Eur J Clin Nutr.* 50(3):152–58.

Johnston CS, Day CS, Swan PD. (2002 Feb) Postprandial thermogenesis is increased

References

100% on a high-protein, low-fat diet versus a high-carbohydrate, low-fat diet in healthy, young women. *J Am Coll Nutr.* 21(1):55–61.

Scalfi L, Coltorti A, Contaldo F. (1991 May) Postprandial thermogenesis in lean and obese subjects after meals supplemented with medium-chain and long-chain triglycerides. *Am J Clin Nutr.* 53(5):1130–33.

Seaton TB, Welle SL, Warenko MK, Campbell RG. (1986 Nov) Thermic effect of medium-chain and long-chain triglycerides in man. *Am J Clin Nutr.* 44(5):630–34.

Soenen S, et al. (2013 May) Normal protein intake is required for body weight loss and weight maintenance, and elevated protein intake for additional preservation of resting energy expenditure and fat free mass. *J Nutr.* 143(5):591–96. doi: 10.3945/jn.112.167593. Epub 2013 Feb 27.

Weickert MO, Pfeiffer AF. (2008 Mar) Metabolic effects of dietary fiber consumption and prevention of diabetes. *J Nutr.* 138(3):439–42.

INCREASED SATIETY

Blom WA, et al. (2006 Feb) Effect of a high-protein breakfast on the postprandial ghrelin response. *Am J Clin Nutr.* 83(2):211–20.

Brennan AM, Sweeney LL, Liu X, Mantzoros CS. (2010 Jun) Walnut consumption increases satiation but has no effect on insulin resistance or the metabolic profile over a 4-day period. *Obesity* (Silver Spring). 18(6):1176–82. doi: 10.1038/oby.2009.409. Epub 2009 Nov 12.

MaÐkowiak K, TorliÐska-Walkowiak N, TorliÐska B. (2016 Feb 25) Dietary fibre as an important constituent of the diet. *Postepy Hig Med Dosw* (Online).70:104–9. doi: 10.5604/17322693.1195842.

Ohlsson B, Höglund P, Roth B, Darwiche G. (2016 Apr) Modification of a traditional breakfast leads to increased satiety along with attenuated plasma increments of glucose, C-peptide, insulin, and glucose-dependent insulinotropic polypeptide in humans. *Nutr Res.* 36(4):359–68. doi: 10.1016/j.nutres.2015.12.004. Epub 2015 Dec 8.

Pal S, Ellis V. (2010 Oct) The acute effects of four protein meals on insulin, glucose, appetite and energy intake in lean men. *Br J Nutr.* 104(8):1241–48. doi: 10.1017/S0007114510001911. Epub 2010 May 11.

Pannacciulli N, et al. (2006 Sep) Higher fasting plasma concentrations of glucagon-like peptide 1 are associated with higher resting energy expenditure and fat oxidation rates in humans. *Am J Clin Nutr.* 84(3):556–60.

Wanders AJ, et al. (2011 Sep). Effects of dietary fibre on subjective appetite, energy intake and body weight: a systematic review of randomized controlled trials. *Obes Rev.* 12(9):724–39. doi: 10.1111/j.1467–789X.2011.00895.x. Epub 2011 Jun 16.

WEIGHT LOSS

Aleixandre A, Miguel M. (2016 Apr) Dietary fiber and blood pressure control. *Food Funct.* 7(4):1864–71. doi: 10.1039/c5fo00950b.

Assunção ML, Ferreira HS, dos Santos AF, Cabral CR Jr, Florêncio TM. (2009 Jul) Effects of dietary coconut oil on the biochemical and anthropometric profiles of women presenting abdominal obesity. *Lipids.* 44(7):593–601. doi: 10.1007/s11745 -009-3306-6. Epub 2009 May 13.

Halkjaer J, et al. (2006 Oct) Intake of macronutrients as predictors of 5-y changes in waist circumference. *Am J Clin Nutr.* 84(4):789–97.

Hariom Y, et al. (2013 Aug 30) Beneficial metabolic effects of a probiotic via butyrate-induced GLP-1 hormone secretion. *J Biol Chem.* 288(35): 25088–97. Published online 2013 Jul 8. doi: 10.1074/jbc.M113.452516 PMCID: PMC3757173.

Liau KM, Lee YY, Chen CK, Rasool AHG. (2011) An open-label pilot study to assess the efficacy and safety of virgin coconut oil in reducing visceral adiposity. *ISRN Pharmacol.* 2011: 949686. Published online 2011 Mar 15. doi: 10.5402/2011/949686 PMCID: PMC3226242.

Layman DK, et al. (2003 Feb) A reduced ratio of dietary carbohydrate to protein improves body composition and blood lipid profiles during weight loss in adult women. *J Nutr.* 133(2):411–17.

Loenneke JP[1], Wilson JM, Manninen AH, Wray ME, Barnes JT, Pujol TJ. (2012 Jan 27) Quality protein intake is inversely related with abdominal fat. *Nutr Metab* (Lond). 9(1):5. doi: 10.1186/1743–7075-9-5.

Pesta D and Samuel VT. (2014) A high-protein diet for reducing body fat: mechanisms and possible caveats. *Nutr Metab* (Lond). 11: 53. Published online 2014 Nov 19. doi: 10.1186/1743–7075-11–53 PMCID: PMC4258944.

Soenen S, et al. (2013 May) Normal protein intake is required for body weight loss and weight maintenance, and elevated protein intake for additional preservation of resting energy expenditure and fat free mass. *J Nutr.* 143(5):591–6. doi: 10.3945 /jn.112.167593. Epub 2013 Feb 27.

REDUCED HUNGER

Crowder CM, Neumann BL, Baum JI. (2016). Breakfast protein source does not influence postprandial appetite response and food intake in normal weight and overweight young women. *J Nutr Metab.* 2016: 6265789. Published online 2016 Jan 17. doi: 10.1155/2016/6265789 PMCID: PMC4739264.

THICKER HAIR

Finner AM. (2013 Jan) Nutrition and hair: deficiencies and supplements. *Dermatol Clin.* 31(1):167–72. doi: 10.1016/j.det.2012.08.015. Epub 2012 Oct 18.

Rizer RL, et al. (2015 Oct–Dec) A marine protein-based dietary supplement for subclinical hair thinning/loss: results of a multisite, double-blind, placebo-controlled clinical trial. *Int J Trichology.* 7(4):156–66. doi: 10.4103/0974–7753.171573.

CLEAR UP SKIN

James MJ, Gibson RA, Cleland LG. (2000 Jan) Dietary polyunsaturated fatty acids and inflammatory mediator production. *Am J Clin Nutr.* 71(1 Suppl):343S–48S.

Meksiarun P, et al. (2015 Jun 21) Analysis of the effects of dietary fat on body and skin lipids of hamsters by Raman spectroscopy. *Analyst.* 140(12):4238–44. doi: 10.1039/c5an00076a. Epub 2015 Apr 29.

SUPPORT IMMUNITY AND FIGHT DISEASE AND INFLAMMATION

Colpo E, et al. (2014 Apr) Brazilian nut consumption by healthy volunteers improves inflammatory parameters. *Nutrition.* 30(4):459–65. doi: 10.1016/j.nut.2013.10.005. Epub 2013 Oct 14.

Grosso G, Estruch R. (2016 Feb) Nut consumption and age-related disease. *Maturitas.* 84:11–16. doi: 10.1016/j.maturitas.2015.10.014. Epub 2015 Nov 2.

Gulati S, et al. (2014 Feb) Effects of pistachio nuts on body composition, metabolic, inflammatory and oxidative stress parameters in Asian Indians with metabolic syndrome: a 24-wk, randomized control trial. *Nutrition.* 30(2):192–97. doi: 10.1016/j.nut.2013.08.005.

James MJ, Gibson RA, Cleland LG. Dietary polyunsaturated fatty acids and inflammatory mediator production. Retrieved from https://www.ncbi.nlm.nih.gov/pubmed/24811150.

Martínez-Cruz O, Paredes-López O. (2014 Jun 13) Phytochemical profile and nutraceutical potential of chia seeds (Salvia hispanica L.) by ultra high performance liquid chromatography. *J Chromatogr A.* 1346:43–48. doi: 10.1016/j.chroma.2014.04.007. Epub 2014 Apr 13.

Nishi SK, et al. (2014 Aug) Nut consumption, serum fatty acid profile and estimated coronary heart disease risk in type 2 diabetes. *Nutr Metab Cardiovasc Dis.* 24(8):845–52. doi: 10.1016/j.numecd.2014.04.001. Epub 2014 May 13.

Parker B, Noakes M, Luscombe N, Clifton P. (2002 Mar) Effect of a high-protein, high-monounsaturated fat weight loss diet on glycemic control and lipid levels in type 2 diabetes. *Diabetes Care.* 25(3):425–30.

Shaik-Dasthagirisaheb YB, et al. (2013 Apr–Jun) Role of vitamins D, E and C in immunity and inflammation. *J Biol Regul Homeost Agents.* 27(2):291–95.

Vuksan V, et al. (2007 Nov) Supplementation of conventional therapy with the novel grain Salba (Salvia hispanica L.) improves major and emerging cardiovascular risk factors in type 2 diabetes: results of a randomized controlled trial. *Diabetes Care.* 30(11):2804–10. Epub 2007 Aug 8.

BETTER SLEEP

De Bernardi Rodrigues AM, et al. (2016 May 1) Association of sleep deprivation with reduction in insulin sensitivity as assessed by the hyperglycemic clamp technique in adolescents. Brazilian Metabolic Syndrome Study (BRAMS) Investigators. *JAMA Pediatr.* 170(5):487–94. doi: 10.1001/jamapediatrics.2015.4365.

Donga E, et al. (2010 Jun) A single night of partial sleep deprivation induces insulin resistance in multiple metabolic pathways in healthy subjects. *J Clin Endocrinol Metab.* 95(6):2963–68. doi: 10.1210/jc.2009–2430. Epub 2010 Apr 6.

Hansen AL, et al. (2014 May 15) Fish consumption, sleep, daily functioning, and heart rate variability. *J Clin Sleep Med.* 10(5): 567–75. Published online 2014 May 15. doi: 10.5664/jcsm.3714 PMCID: PMC4013386.

Montgomery P, et al. (2014 Aug). Fatty acids and sleep in UK children: subjective and pilot objective sleep results from the DOLAB study—a randomized controlled trial. *J Sleep Res.* 23(4):364–88. doi:10.1111/jsr.12135. Epub 2014 Mar 8.

MENTAL CLARITY

Bourre JM. (2004 Sep). [The role of nutritional factors on the structure and function of the brain: an update on dietary requirements]. [Article in French] *Rev Neurol* (Paris). 160(8–9):767–92.

——. (2004) Roles of unsaturated fatty acids (especially omega-3 fatty acids) in the brain at various ages and during ageing. *J Nutr Health Aging.* 8(3):163–74.

——. (2006 Sep-Oct). Effects of nutrients (in food) on the structure and function of the nervous system: update on dietary requirements for brain. Part 2: macronutrients. *J Nutr Health Aging.* 10(5):386–99.

References

——. (2006 Sep-Oct). Effects of nutrients (in food) on the structure and function of the nervous system: update on dietary requirements for brain. Part 1: micronutrients. *J Nutr Health Aging.* 10(5):377–85.

Crowder CM, Neumann BL, Baum JI. (2016) Breakfast protein source does not influence postprandial appetite response and food intake in normal weight and overweight young women. *J Nutr Metab.* 2016: 6265789. Published online 2016 Jan 17. doi: 10.1155/2016/6265789 PMCID: PMC4739264.

Leidy HJ, Ortinau LC, Douglas SM, Hoertel HA. (2013 Apr) Beneficial effects of a higher-protein breakfast on the appetitive, hormonal, and neural signals controlling energy intake regulation in overweight/obese, "breakfast-skipping," late-adolescent girls. *Am J Clin Nutr.* 97(4):677–88. doi: 10.3945/ajcn.112.053116. Epub 2013 Feb 27.

Tangney CC, et al. (2011 Sep 27) Vitamin B12, cognition, and brain MRI measures: a cross-sectional examination. *Neurology.* 77(13):1276–82. doi: 10.1212/WNL.0b013e3182315a33.

INCREASED LEAN MUSCLE MASS

Cheng B, et al. (1997 May) Time course of the effects of a high-fat diet and voluntary exercise on muscle enzyme activity in Long-Evans rats. *Physiol Behav.* 61(5):701–5.

Hector AJ, et al. (2015 Feb) Whey protein supplementation preserves postprandial myofibrillar protein synthesis during short-term energy restriction in overweight and obese adults. *J Nutr.* 145(2):246–52. doi: 10.3945/jn.114.200832. Epub 2014 Dec 17.

Hulmi JJ, Lockwood CM, Stout JR. (2010 Jun 17) Effect of protein/essential amino acids and resistance training on skeletal muscle hypertrophy: A case for whey protein. *Nutr Metab* (Lond). 7:51. doi: 10.1186/1743–7075-7-51.

Li X, Higashida K, Kawamura T, Higuchi M. (2016 Apr 6). Alternate-day high-fat diet induces an increase in mitochondrial enzyme activities and protein content in rat skeletal muscle. *Nutrients.* 8(4):203. doi: 10.3390/nu8040203.

Loenneke JP, Loprinzi PD, Murphy CH, Phillips SM. (2016 Apr 7) Per meal dose and frequency of protein consumption is associated with lean mass and muscle performance. *Clin Nutr.* 35(6):1506–1. doi: 10.1016/j.clnu.2016.04.002.

Pasiakos SM, McLellan TM, Lieberman HR. (2015 Jan) The effects of protein supplements on muscle mass, strength, and aerobic and anaerobic power in healthy adults: a systematic review. *Sports Med.* 45(1):111–31. doi: 10.1007/s40279-014-0242-2.

UNIVERSAL CONVERSION CHART

OVEN TEMPERATURE EQUIVALENTS

$250°F = 120°C$ $\qquad$ $400°F = 200°C$

$275°F = 135°C$ $\qquad$ $425°F = 220°C$

$300°F = 150°C$ $\qquad$ $450°F = 230°C$

$325°F = 160°C$ $\qquad$ $475°F = 240°C$

$350°F = 180°C$ $\qquad$ $500°F = 260°C$

$375°F = 190°C$

MEASUREMENT EQUIVALENTS

Measurements should always be level unless directed otherwise.

$\frac{1}{8}$ teaspoon	=	0.5 ml			
$\frac{1}{4}$ teaspoon	=	1 ml			
$\frac{1}{2}$ teaspoon	=	2 ml			
1 teaspoon	=	5 ml			
1 tablespoon	=	3 teaspoons	= $\frac{1}{2}$ fluid ounce	=	15 mL
2 tablespoons	=	$\frac{1}{8}$ cup	= 1 fluid ounce	=	30 mL
4 tablespoons	=	$\frac{1}{4}$ cup	= 2 fluid ounces	=	60 mL
$5\frac{1}{3}$ tablespoons	=	$\frac{1}{3}$ cup	= 3 fluid ounces	=	80 mL
8 tablespoons	=	$\frac{1}{2}$ cup	= 4 fluid ounces	=	120 mL
$10\frac{2}{3}$ tablespoons	=	$\frac{2}{3}$ cup	= 5 fluid ounces	=	160 mL
12 tablespoons	=	$\frac{3}{4}$ cup	= 6 fluid ounces	=	180 mL
16 tablespoons	=	1 cup	= 8 fluid ounces	=	240 mL

UNIVERSAL CONVERSION CHART

ACKNOWLEDGMENTS

A very special thank-you to my first-ever-book team—my wise and wonderful agent, Yfat Reiss Gendell, my trusted and lovely writing partner, Billie Fitzpatrick, and my husband, Chris, who always has my back. This book would not have happened without all of you.

To my amazing team at Morrow: Thanks especially to editor extraordinaire Cassie Jones, and to Kara Zauberman, Anwesha Basu, Molly Waxman, Andrew DiCecco, Bonni Leon-Berman, and Serena Wang. I am so grateful for their help shepherding *Body Love* to fruition.

To my creative team, photographer Vanessa Tierney and graphic designer Amber Moon, thank you for bringing *Body Love* to life with color, imagery, and art.

A special thank-you to my family—my parents and sisters, whose unwavering support of me and belief in me and my dreams have made them come true with this book.

And a *huge* thank-you to all my clients for trusting me with their health and happiness. Their inspiration and experience has truly brought *Body Love* alive. Without them, my practice would simply not exist.

INDEX

Index

Index

Index

Index

Index

Index